Jacques Lacan and
the Adventure of Insight

Jacques Lacan and the Adventure of Insight

Psychoanalysis in Contemporary Culture

Shoshana Felman

Harvard University Press
Cambridge, Massachusetts
and London, England

Permission to use quotations from the works of Lacan has been granted
by Editions du Seuil and by Jacques-Alain Miller, "exécuteur testamentaire
de Jacques Lacan et dépositaire du droit moral sur son oeuvre."

Library of Congress Cataloging-in-Publication Data

Felman, Shoshana.
   Jacques Lacan and the adventure of insight.

   Bibliography: p.
   1. Psychoanalysis and literature.   2. Criticism.
3. Lacan, Jacques, 1901–1981—Contributions in
criticism.   I. Title.
PN98.P75F45   1987   801'.92   86-19458
ISBN 0-674-47120-2 (alk. paper) (cloth)
ISBN 0-674-47121-0 (paper)

This book has been digitally reprinted. The content
remains identical to that of previous printings.

For my students

Can we now perhaps find the place where strangeness was present, the place where a person succeeded in setting himself free? ... Perhaps at this point is an Other set free?

Paul Celan

Acknowledgments

■ This book was written in the condition of a constant dialogue with friends, whom I would like to take this opportunity to thank:

First of all, Barbara Johnson, who enriched me with her insight and afforded me critical perspective in patiently accompanying me through the pages of this book.

My editors: Lindsay Waters, who supported me through the stimulating and responsive interest he took in the creation—and completion—of this book; Joyce Backman, who spared neither time nor effort in trying to add clarity and cogency to the manuscript.

Nathaniel Laor, M.D., Dori Laub, M.D., Darius Ornston, M.D., John Muller, and Miri Kubovi, the other companions of various moments of my writing, who read parts of the manuscript and contributed to it the resonances of their understanding and the improvements of their perspicacious criticism.

And Tom Pepper, who with meticulous and caring attention saw the page proofs through final correction.

■ Chapter 2, "The Case of Poe," was first published under the title "On Reading Poetry: Reflections on the Limits and Possibilities of Psychoanalytical Approaches," in *The Literary Freud: Mechanisms of Defense and the Poetic Will,* edited by J. H. Smith (New Haven: Yale University Press, 1980). A first version of Chapter 3, "What Difference Does Psychoanalysis Make? or The Originality of Freud," was published in *Poetics Today* ("Theory: Modern Trends"), vol. 2, no. 1b (Winter 1980–1981). A first version of Chapter 4, "Psychoanalysis and Education: Teaching Terminable and Interminable," was published in *Yale French Studies,* no. 63 1 (The Pedagogical Imperative), edited by Barbara Johnson (New Haven: Yale University Press, 1982). The second half of Chapter 5, "Beyond Oedipus: The Specimen Story of Psychoanalysis," was published, under the same title, in *MLN* (Baltimore, The Johns Hopkins University), vol. 98, no. 5 (December 1983).

Contents

All I can do is tell the truth. No, that isn't so—I have missed it. There is no truth that, in passing through awareness, does not lie.   But one runs after it all the same.

Lacan, *The Four Fundamental Concepts of Psychoanalysis*

INTRODUCTION ■

An Act That Is
Yet To Come

■ I will start by recounting the peculiar story of my first encounter with Lacan's work. Though it may sound like mere anecdote, I think it is an anecdote worth sharing, since it exemplifies a dramatically instructive way of encountering the significance of Lacan. Furthermore, the peculiar way in which Lacan has come across my path, the specific manner in which his work came to appeal to me, is singularly telling, I believe, about one of the ways in which thought can be experienced today.

■ Between Theory and Practice: My Encounter with Lacan

I was a student in a European university, working on a Ph.D. in literature. Jacques Lacan was, at that time, heatedly polemicized and discussed among the French intelligentsia.[1] I first heard Lacan's name mentioned by two highly respected teachers in the university. One of them kept referring to Lacan with enthusiasm and admiration. The other would mention Lacan in a derogatory way, advising us, in sum, not to read him. I was struck both by the contradiction and by the fact that there could be something that a teacher would teach us not to learn. I became curious and decided to read Lacan's book (there was only one published at the time, the *Ecrits*). I went to the university bookstore, picked up the volume, and took it to the cashier, who was also the store's owner.

To my surprise, the man advised me not to buy the book. "Why?" I asked. "Aren't you in the business of selling books?" "Yes," he answered, "but I am also here to give advice to students: this is an expensive book, and I promise you: it is unreadable, totally incomprehensible. Don't buy it."

Thus began the process of apprenticeship through which I came to know Lacan's work.

Jacques Lacan is without doubt one of the most influential and controversial French thinkers of this century. In the history of psychoanalysis, indeed, his capacity to inspire both passionate agreement and passionate disagreement has been matched only by Freud's. His iconoclastic impact is at once outstanding and unsettling. How can one comprehend a figure with such a record of controversiality? With a few exceptions, most attempts to understand Lacan have assumed the shape either of a didactic exposition of Lacan's complicated thought or of a polemical defense of Lacan's position in the context of the controversy among different psychoanalytic factions.

I will pursue another path, in an attempt to achieve a clarification of another kind: I will neither explicate Lacan as a set of foreclosed conceptual dogmas, nor will I engage in a debate about his controversial personality. Instead I will attempt to share here with the reader the lived experience of a discovery: of the discovery that psychoanalysis has opened up for me through my encounter with Lacan's work. I propose to explore, in the pages that will follow, at once the insights that I have obtained from working with Lacan's text and the way those insights have made a difference in my own relation both to life and to my work.

The very fact that I have started by telling you a story, to which I will return, the fact that in this introduction I will from time to time address the reader as "you" while referring to my own voice as "I," itself partakes of a question that is meaningful with respect to crucial analytic issues that Lacan is specifically concerned with: issues such as dialogue and the performative psychoanalytic character of understanding and of knowledge as itself an act, a process of narration. It should be understood, however, that the pronouns "I" and "you" are not merely personal but also metaphorical or allegorical. If "I" and "you" are here, in practice, a pragmatic entryway into a theoretical (analytic) problematics, what they talk about should be approached with caution. As Lacan puts it,

> It is not a question of knowing whether I speak of myself in a way that conforms to what I am, but rather of knowing whether I am the same as that of which I speak. (E, N 165)[2]

Let me get back to the story. In spite of the advice that I was offered not to buy and not to read Lacan's work, I did end up buying the book and reading it. My paradoxical advantage in this reading was that, being an outsider to the psychoanalytic field, I knew very little of the polemical passions and institutional quarrels around Lacan. More important, being neither an analyst nor an analysand, I did not care whether or not I understood the book. I did not *have* to understand it: I did not have to prove anything or to be accountable to anyone for my reading. Working at the time on my literary dissertation, I was merely interested in seeing for myself if this text had anything to offer me. I simply read through it, without fighting with it, without trying to appropriate it as a piece of academic information.

A great number of the pages I was reading did in fact seem incomprehensible, but at the same time they profoundly moved me. Lacan's writing read like Mallarmé's—an obscure and enigmatic, yet powerful and effective, poetic prose.[3] It appealed to me in the way literature appeals to me: without my being able to make immediate sense of it or translate it, I was made to take in and absorb more than I knew.

What I later realized was that my reading of Lacan was radically transforming my own writing, my dissertation on Stendhal.[4] My writing was transformed not, however, in the sense that I tried to imitate Lacan's idiomatic style, but in the sense that I began to read the literature I was working on in an altogether different manner: suddenly having insights into textual details in Stendhal's work that I had simply failed to notice, to perceive as significant, before.

As Lacan became a tool for my enhanced literary understanding, what he enabled me to understand from literature was enabling me in turn, over the years, to read him better, to gain clearer insight into his own work. So, in the pursuit of my own literary work and concurrently of my reading of Lacan, each was teaching me how to read the other.

My first encounter with Lacan's work had, in that way, taken place from within the field of literature, outside the domain of psychoanalysis proper. My acquaintance with Lacan—and through him with psychoanalysis—was thus mostly theoretical at first. But I had the shock of an encounter with the Lacanian experience a second time—in quite a different manner—when I became, years later in the United States, an analysand myself.

My analyst did not belong to any Lacanian persuasion: he was, in fact, quite unfamiliar with Lacan. And yet his clinical behavior and his therapeutic stance put into effect, and underscored, the crucial clinical features that Lacan's theory was focused on.[5]

I was struck by this coincidence: I was witnessing the metamorphosis of my aesthetic/intellectual involvement with a theory into the surprising lived experience—the compelling eloquence—of a clinical event that resonated with it. It was then that for the first time I could see not merely the sheer intellectual luxury—the subtlety of insight—of Lacan's theory, but its more concrete dimension of unexpected efficacy, of clinical inevitability.

It came to me as a surprising new discovery how much Lacan's familiar theoretical considerations were focused on—committed to and totally immersed in—the very matrix of the clinical experience, of psychoanalysis as a singular event rather than as pure cognition; and how much the basic truths of the clinical experience, the basic insights into clinical experience (into an effective clinical positioning of the psychoanalytic stance), were in fact in line with what Lacan was emphasizing, differences in theoretical outlook notwithstanding. It seemed now that Lacan's work was encountering and making more complex the insight gained from my own analysis, whereas my analysis was shifting my perspective on Lacan.

I realized that Lacan was first and foremost a clinician, and not—as is mistakenly believed and as the myth would have it—a pure theoretician. Though fascinated by new scientific models challenging the mind—challenging the habits and breaking the routines—of the established cognitive and intellectual imagination, Lacan's elaborate conceptual framework in effect is trying to describe, most simply and most fundamentally, why and how the practice *works;* why and how, in the structured Freudian analytic setting, something like a clinical experience comes about: takes hold and takes effect.

Contrary to popular opinion, what matters most in Lacan's clinical conception is not his technical, eccentric innovations: the controversial short session, for example, does not deserve the centrality the controversy has given it. The concept of a possibly shortened session emphasizes the relationship between treatment and time and between interpretation and punctuation, offering to make of the punctuation—the ending of the session—a *variable* interpretation, which might accelerate and stimulate the session's productivity, underscore high points, and perhaps be an auxiliary in the working through of separations and temporal discontinuities. But this experimental change was mainly arguing for the pragmatic possibility of an open-minded and intelligent flexibility with regard to clinical conventions, rather than claiming to be a major theoretical contribution or an indispensable, dogmatic innovation.

What I learned to understand from my own analytical experience, then, is that Lacan's true clinical originality consists not in the incidental innovations that separate his theory from other schools, but in the insight he gives us, paradoxically enough, into the very structural foundations of what is in practice *common to all schools:* in his uniquely sharp clinical grasp and his strikingly original account of the transference relation and of the dialogic psychoanalytic situation, insofar as those two key principles of therapeutic action operate, in fact, within each psychoanalytic theoretical orientation.

This shifting perspective on Lacan, and the growing awareness of the primacy of practice over theory that my own analysis set in motion, corresponds in turn to a shifting relation between theory and practice in my own life. Since I have gone through a period of training at a psychoanalytic institute, I have come to a deeper understanding of how theory and practice on the one hand, psychoanalysis and literature on the other, keep informing and, in fact, training each other.

■ Lacan as Metaphor, or the Subject of the Book

There are at least two possible approaches to the description of an intellectual figure. One is to describe the figure from outside, to assess its value or significance on the basis of a comparison with other figures. Another choice is to describe the figure from inside, to enter its own world, to participate in the momentum of its own internal movement in an attempt to grasp the inner thrust of its originality. This second manner is the one I have chosen in this book.[6]

Such an approach may seem at moments to imply the preclusion of other figures and achievements in the field of psychoanalysis, as if Lacan's were the best possible or the sole worthwhile approach to psychoanalytic insight. This is obviously not so. I am well aware of the fact that the wealth of the field of psychoanalysis comprises other theoretical perspectives and practical decisions. But the thrust of my attempt is to explore Lacan in his own terms: to reach as deep as one can reach into Lacan's own frame of reference. Far from claiming that this frame of reference stands for the only valid or the most legitimate conception, my empathic stance—my intellectual adherence to this frame—is one of searching for the usefulness, the productivity, the creativity inherent in it: it seeks to derive and to explore the utmost *inspiration* that this frame of reference might be capable of yielding.

Inasmuch as this inspiration goes beyond the literality of the frame of reference (defying and evading its dogmatic grasp), my subject is necessarily larger than Lacan: it is the cultural fecundity of psychoanalysis, the general significance of psychoanalysis for contemporary culture. Lacan is a convenient tool for understanding this significance, since he specifically attempts to understand and to restate the momentousness of Freud's discovery in contemporary terms. Whereas Freud articulated his discovery through a metaphoric use of the conceptual framework of nineteenth-century science (thermodynamics, topology, and such), Lacan has tried to instrumentalize for psychoanalysis some twentieth-century theoretical and scientific findings. Borrowing paradigmatic (metaphoric) models from linguistics, anthropology, philosophy, symbolic logic, cybernetics, modern physics, mathematics (set theory), and topology (knot theory), Lacan attempts to integrate the conceptual import of these models into psychoanalytic theory and to rethink the cognitive revolution of psychoanalysis along the lines of other recent revolutionary theories.

Lacan's endeavor can itself be read, then, as a metaphor (or perhaps a symptom) of the cognitive revolution brought about by psychoanalysis, insofar as Lacan is a reminder of the fact that this revolution has affected all areas of our cultural life, in ways whose implications are still disquietingly unpredictable. Lacan is thus a metaphor—or a symptom—of psychoanalysis itself, insofar as psychoanalysis is reenacting a constant revolution in the most basic human questions:

What does it mean to be human?

What does it mean to think? and consequently,

What does it mean to be contemporary?[7]

This is, in Lacan's perspective, what the revolution called psychoanalysis is forcing us to question and requestion. And this is, in effect, the real subject of my book.

The book, in other words, is perhaps less about Lacan than it is about a contemporary way of reading that psychoanalysis has made possible: a way of reading I have learned from Lacan, and which my reading of him on one level constantly enacts (puts into effect, plays out) while, on another level, it attempts to analyze it and account for its difference. Lacan indeed embodies in my view, above all else, a revolutionized interpretive stance and (though he never formulates it systematically) a revolutionary theory of reading: a theory of reading that opens up into a rereading of the world as well as into a rereading of psychoanalysis itself.

Lacan is thus a figure in my book of the simple fact that the last word of psychoanalysis (or on psychoanalysis) has not yet been said: the figure of an opening, an interminability, some unfinished business, emerging at the not yet understood horizon of psychoanalysis. Lacan invites us to a rediscovery of Freud as a profoundly renewed and profoundly unsettling intellectual adventure. But this adventure is composed not only of the momentum of the process of discovery but also of the revolution started by psychoanalysis, and of the challenge to psychoanalysis that this ongoing revolution necessarily contains within itself. Lacan embodies, and is here a metaphor for, both.

■ The Structure of the Book

Let me now sketch out my general conception of the book and outline its chapters.

Chapter 1, "Renewing the Practice of Reading," describes psychoanalysis as, primarily, a revolutionary lesson of reading. Through Freud and through Lacan, I attempt to address the general question: How does psychoanalytic insight modify both the interpretive stance and the very conception of the basic cultural act of reading (and of writing)?

Chapters 2 and 5 (on Poe and Oedipus) include Lacanian psychoanalytic readings and the way in which those specific readings open up into a rereading of the fundamental structures of psychoanalysis, thus having general theoretical and methodological consequences. The practical readings are, indeed, exemplary of Lacan's procedure (of Lacan's lesson of reading) not just in that they amount to original theoretical conclusions, but also in that each pragmatic reading always has a *triple* reference: a reference to a literary text, which it is specifically interpreting; a reference to a text by Freud, with which it is specifically interpreting; and a reference to clinical practice, for which Freud's text is trying to account, and of which the literary text is always in some way a telling paradigm, a metaphorical dramatization.

Chapter 2, "The Case of Poe," gives an example of such a Lacanian reading in outlining, first, the difference between traditional psychoanalytic interpretations of Poe and Lacan's radically different approach in his interpretation of Poe's tale, "The Purloined Letter." What is at stake in this chapter, however, goes far beyond Poe and exceeds as well the didactic question of the methodologies with which psychoanalysis can interpret literature. If I am using literature here as a starting point, it is not simply because literature happens to be my field but because literature is a convenient ground on which a sharper, vaster, and more urgent question can be raised: the crucial question of the use-value of psychoanalysis (in what conditions is psychoanalysis usable?); the question of the very possibility of *application* of psychoanalytic knowledge, not just outside psychoanalysis but within the psychoanalytic treatment as well.

Psychoanalysts know well from their clinical practice that there are no simple applications of psychoanalytic concepts. In practice (as a therapist or as a reader, a literary critic), one can use theories (as I am here trying to use Lacan and Freud) only as enabling metaphorical devices, not as extrapolated, preconceived items of knowledge. In much the same way that one cannot simply "apply" Freud's concepts to a patient, one cannot apply Freud (or Lacan) to a literary text. The practice of psychoanalysis (as well as the experience of a practical reading) is a process, not a set of doctrines. In the process, one can *implicate* the doctrines, one can perhaps imply them, not apply them.[8]

Poe's "Purloined Letter" is a case in point, since it provides us, in Lacan's perspective, with a dramatic allegory of psychoanalysis. On the basis of this allegory, I want to argue that psychoanalytic knowledge (Freud's theory, Lacan's theory, or whatever) is itself necessarily a purloined (lost, displaced, or misplaced) letter: it is never simply there, at our disposal to apply. It is something that we necessarily keep losing and have to keep working at to find again. But we cannot find it (have it) once and for all. Like the purloined letter, *psychoanalysis always has to be recovered.*

And this is what Lacan, in fact, is all about: about the necessary loss of psychoanalysis, and about its possible recovery, but only on the condition that it never be taken for granted. Above all else, clinicians, in Lacan's view, must never take themselves for granted: they must never take for granted (be complacent with) their own "ego"; must not confuse this ego with the title and authority with which they can become endowed by virtue of the structure of the therapeutic situation.

Lacan's clinical emphasis calls out for a therapeutic self-efface-ment of the clinician's ego (for a clinical suspicion, with respect to the clinician's unavoidable idealized self-image, which should be kept in check, outside the picture of the therapeutic drama). This clinical guideline can be best understood in the context of Lacan's particular theory of the ego. As distinct from other psychoanalytic theories of the ego, for Lacan the ego is not an autonomous syn-thetic function of the subject, but only the delusion of such a function. The outcome of a series of narcissistic identifications, the ego is the mirror structure of an imaginary, self-idealizing *self-alienation of the subject.* It is a structure of denial: denial of cas-tration (through a unified self-aggrandizement) and denial of sub-jectivity (through objectification of others and self-objectification). As such, the ego, in Lacan's conception, cannot be the origin of any cure or the reference point for the therapeutic alliance. The ego, says Lacan, is itself "structured like a symptom . . . Inside the subject, it is nothing other than a privileged symptom. It is the human symptom par excellence. The ego is human being's mental illness" (S 1.22). Therefore the ego of the analyst must not be taken as the clinical criterion for reality, normality, or health, and should thus serve neither as a model for the development of a strong autonomous ego in the patient nor as a reference point for a cure effected through narcissistic identification. Through Poe's story, Lacan shows how the analyst's effectiveness proceeds not from the superiority of his/her knowledge, gifts, perception of reality, or moral ideology, but from the analyst's position in a symbolic structure that repeats itself: the structure of the clinical situation, insofar as it repeats and picks up on the symbolic (as opposed to the imaginary) structure of the unconscious of the patient.

Chapter 3, "What Difference Does Psychoanalysis Make? or The Originality of Lacan," attempts to synthesize Lacan's perspective on the originality of the very discipline of psychoanalysis. This originality is, for Lacan, the outcome not just of Freud's thought but of its process. Freudian insight, Lacan claims, is not a cognitive possession, it is an event: the singular event of a discovery, the unique advent of a moment of illumination that, because it cannot by its very nature become a heritage, an acquisition, has to be repeated, reenacted, practiced each time for the first time.

Lacan's endeavor is thus not so much to innovate as to probe the nature of the *ineradicable newness* of Freud's insight. By analyzing the significance of Lacan's way of making Freud's thought new again, and of thus enabling us to participate in the very moment of intellectual struggle and illumination, I want to show in what way this moment of illumination has become crucial to contemporary thinking and has *redefined insight as such.* The chapter thus attempts to address the questions: What has happened to thinking after Freud? What kind of scientific thinking has the Freudian discovery opened up, and what kind of thinking has it precluded? How does psychoanalysis, though radically different from philosophy, nonetheless define a new model of rationality?

Chapter 4, "Psychoanalysis and Education," explores what I take to be the potential (but as yet mostly misconstrued) psychoanalytic contribution to theories of education. How does psychoanalysis transform the traditional conception of knowledge and its transmission? What is the significance of transference for teaching? How should the psychoanalytic process of knowing and learning inform and modify the classroom situation?

Lacan's unusual style and his unusual practice as a teacher, his conflation of the interminability of didactic analysis with education in a self-reflexive and self-questioning process of teaching, which makes a pedagogical imperative of its own refusal to take itself (its own authority) for granted, may suggest a revolutionary psychoanalytic lesson about lessons. It is up to us, however, to derive this lesson for ourselves. It is up to us to participate—as students, teachers, analysts, analysands, or readers—in the pedagogical adventure of the psychoanalytic insight whose last word, precisely, has not yet been said.

My own translation of Lacan's performative, though unarticulated, pedagogical lesson was worked out through my own practice of teaching. And, in fact, many of the lessons of this book originated in the freshness, the responsiveness, the engaging insight of my students: those who, in particular, have taken part in my seminar on Lacan.

Chapter 5, "Beyond Oedipus," is the culmination of the volume. Of all the chapters here, it is the most recent, with the exception of this introduction. It is therefore the piece that goes farthest along the intellectual and biographical itinerary I have been trying to sketch out. It is, specifically, the chapter that is most concerned with what can be listened to, and heard, within and out of the pragmatics of a setting that is clinical, the piece that is the most involved with the clinical experience in itself and from within itself, attempting to derive and to articulate the basics of Lacan's clinical insights (even though Lacan's discussion of the clinical events analyzed here is by indirection—through the intermediary of his critical reinterpretation of a case report by Melanie Klein).

This final chapter is also, doubtless, the most encompassing account I can give of Lacan's lesson of reading, of Lacan's commitment to the triple reference—his persistent and creative use of the triple dimension of practice (clinical event), concept (theory), and metaphor (literature), in his multilayered and irreducibly complex account of all three together: of the practical teachings of the clinical experience, in their relation to the theoretical teachings of Freud's work, in their relation to the resonances, to the figural teachings, of a specimen literary text.

The chapter includes an elucidation of the Oedipus complex in Lacan's rendering, as the asymmetrically triangular (rather than symmetrically dualistic) symbolic structure constitutive of subjectivity. The triangularity of that structure also accounts for what happens in the clinical set-up and, primarily, in the analytic dialogue, which is only in appearance dual but which becomes effective not by virtue of its illusory specularity (narcissistic, loving mutual reflexion between the ego of the analyst and the ego of the patient) but by virtue of the triangular asymmetry through which the analyst comes to occupy (as in Poe's story) the symbolic position of the unconscious of the patient. In effect, the analyst speaks on the same side as the patient, not opposite the patient.

On the basis of Melanie Klein's case history, understood in light of his own clinical insight and of the insight he concurrently derives from Sophocles' tragedies *(Oedipus the King, Oedipus at Colonus)* and from Freud's earlier and later works *(The Interpretation of Dreams, Beyond the Pleasure Principle)*, Lacan reconstructs the key psychoanalytic concept of the Oedipus complex, not as an answer but as the structure of a question.

Lacan himself must hold just a position in that structure. Our attitude to Lacan, therefore, should remain complex. If I choose to read in this same chapter Lacan's historical exclusion from the International Psychoanalytical Association as another repercussion or reverberation of the psychoanalytic (Oedipal) specimen story, it should be understood that my reading, far from being simply factual, is metaphorical, playing out its own literary resonances and deliberately operating at the level of a parable.

I am arguing essentially not for the rightness of Lacan's position but for its compelling psychoanalytic exemplarity and, through it, for the endless psychoanalytic "narrativity" of understanding. What is at stake, in other words, in my own practical and theoretical lesson of reading, beyond Lacan, is the fact that there is no psychoanalytic understanding that can dispense with narrative or truly go beyond it. It is primarily within the double task this chapter has assigned itself, to understand psychoanalytic narrative and to narrate psychoanalytic understanding, that Lacan becomes a parable: at once a metaphor and a symptom of psychoanalysis itself.

■ The Blindness of Insight, or Thinking Beyond Our Means

If I have related to you not just how I read Lacan but the way in which I came to read him in the way I do, it is because reading, as I see it, is a constant struggle to become aware. Reading is an access route to a discovery. But the significance of the discovery appears only in retrospect, because insight is never purely cognitive; it is to some extent always performative (incorporated in an act, a doing) and to that extent precisely it is not transparent to itself. Insight is always partially unconscious, partially partaking of a practice. And since there can never be a simultaneous, full coincidence between practice and awareness, what one understands in doing and through doing appears in retrospect: *nachträglich, après coup.*

It is now, in retrospect, that I see more clearly the significance of the impact that my discovery of Lacan's work, years ago, has had on me: Lacan has been a major access route to insight. And since the struggle to become aware can never reach a term, the route itself—a route of reading—might be as important as the insight to which it hopes to lead. This is why I have attempted to preface the description of the Lacanian adventure of insight by tracing here my route to his, *and* my route through his.

Since for Lacan psychoanalysis is an invention that, in its practice, *teaches people how to think beyond their means,* I have attempted to follow up on the Lacanian challenge and to read Lacan's own thought (in the way that he himself attempts to read Freud) beyond the limits (and the limitations) of its own awareness. I have attempted, in other words, to articulate and to reach into the significance of Lacan's insight, beyond the literal perception (the dogmatization) of his text, his acts, his practice, and his clinical techniques.

This book, then, is an attempt to explore some of the key possibilities that Lacan has opened up—for psychoanalysis, for culture, and for reading; an attempt to illuminate a way of reading whose unending struggle to become aware was able, in the process, to *become attentive* to messages or items of signification that were formerly unusable and, as such, unreadable, inaudible, invisible. This is, in my view, the quintessential service that Lacan has rendered to our culture: to have derived from Freud a way of reading whose unprecedented thrust and achievement is to keep an entire system of signification open, rather than foreclose it, so that the small, unnoticeable messages can grow, by virtue of the fact that the big ones are kept still, open and suspended. In trying here both to illuminate and to practice this way of reading, I hope not simply to repay a small share of the debt of inspiration Lacan has given me, but to do Lacan, psychoanalysis, and all those who are interested in insight a justice of a different order, by making these creative possibilities, and this access route to insight, a little more *accessible* to all of us—in our theories as well as in our lives.

CHAPTER ONE ■

An Exemplary Lesson of Reading ■
A Theory of Practice ■
Freud as Reader ■
After Freud ■

Renewing the Practice of Reading, or Freud's Unprecedented Lesson

■ I would like to address, in the light of Lacan's radical rethinking of the crucial psychoanalytic issue of interpretation, the general question—both practical and theoretical—of the relationship between psychoanalysis and reading. In theory: What insight does psychoanalysis provide into the very nature of interpretation? In practice: How has psychoanalysis modified the nature and the possibilities of reading by drastically transforming the procedures, strategies, and techniques available to the interpreter?

■ An Exemplary Lesson of Reading

In 1968 the French philosopher Louis Althusser wrote of Lacan:

> It is to the intransigent, lucid—and for many years solitary—theoretical effort of Jacques Lacan that we owe today this result [a new understanding of the mechanisms of the discourse of the unconscious], which has drastically transformed our way of reading Freud. At a time when what Lacan has given us that was so radically new begins to pass into the public domain and when everyone can use it, in his own way, to his profit, I would like to make a point of acknowledging our debt toward his exemplary lesson of reading, the effects of which, as we shall see, go well beyond its original object.[1]

While fully subscribing to Althusser's acknowledgment, I would suggest that we can by no means take it for granted that Lacan's "exemplary lesson of reading" has in any way been *learned*, let alone assimilated, even by those of us who are familiar with his work, those who have been immersed in the (French) public domain that has so eagerly appropriated his concepts and words. A lesson—any lesson—cannot simply be confused with the words, the terminology it uses to articulate itself. A reading lesson is, precisely, not a statement; it is a performance. It is not theory, it is practice, a practice that derives—as such—its worth from its efficiency, not from its exemplarity; a practice, therefore, that can be exemplary only insofar as it is understood to be a model or a paradigm, not for imitation but for (self) transformation. The passage of Lacan's original terminology into the public domain that has indeed appropriated it for a variety of usages and profits, far from ensuring an understanding of the lesson, in effect blocks such understanding, serves itself as a defense against the lesson. For, as was the case with Freud, it is not in words that the lesson can be learned, but in the body, in one's life.

It is true that words are what we read; and in this case we have to read Lacan's words, from which we have to learn how to read. But language for Lacan (even his own) is something altogether other than a list of terms to be mastered. It is rather something like a list of terms we should be transformed by, a list of terms into which to write, or to translate, ourselves.

The American philosopher Richard Rorty writes that "we are in for another few hundred years of getting adjusted to the availability of the psychoanalytic vocabulary."[2] By way of agreeing with this statement, I would suggest that we are in for another few hundred years of getting adjusted to the availability of Lacan's lesson of reading; a lesson that itself is an attempt toward, precisely, the adjustment or translation of our modes of thinking and of operating to the still unassimilated radicality of the Freudian revolution.

In acknowledging my own debt to Lacan's exemplary lesson of reading, I can only try to be a teacher of this lesson insofar as I am its student: I can offer only my own reading of Lacan's unformulated theory of reading, through an analysis of Lacan's practice as a reader and of what constitutes what I take to be the pathbreaking originality of this practice. But this analysis should itself be viewed as but a step in the effort, that is, in the far from finished process, of adjusting my own ways of thinking and of operating (of adjusting my own ways of reading) to the availability of both the Lacanian and the Freudian insights. I will try, in other words, to read Lacan's lesson of reading not just in my statement about what Lacan is doing when he reads, when he articulates a reading, but in my own way of articulating such a statement, in my own practice as reader.

■ A Theory of Practice

What is the relationship between psychoanalysis and reading in Lacan's particular perspective on the matter?

"It is obvious," says Lacan, "that in analytic discourse, what is at stake is nothing other than what can be read; what can be read beyond what the subject has been incited to say" (S xx.29). "What is at stake in analytic discourse is always this—to what is uttered as a signifier [by the patient], you [analysts] give another reading than what it means" (S xx.37). In these two quotations that describe the practice of psychoanalysis, "reading" refers to the analyst's activity of interpreting, and the emphasis is on the displacement operated by the interpreting: the analyst is called upon to interpret the excess in the patient's discourse—what the patient says *beyond* what he has been incited to say, beyond the current motivation of the situation; and the analytic meaning is then a displacement of the meaning of the patient's discourse, since it consists in giving what has been pronounced *another reading*. The analytic reading is thus essentially the reading of a difference that inhabits language, a kind of mapping in the subject's discourse of its points of dis-agreement with, or difference from, itself.

This, however, is still by and large the conventional view of the role of reading in analysis. Lacan's view is more radical than that. For the activity of reading is not just the analyst's, it is also the analysand's: interpreting is what takes place *on both sides* of the analytic situation. The unconscious, in Lacan's eyes, is not simply the object of psychoanalytical investigation, but its subject. The unconscious, in other words, is not simply *that which must be read* but also, and perhaps primarily, *that which reads.* The unconscious is a reader. What this implies most radically is that whoever reads, interprets out of his unconscious, is an analysand, even when the interpreting is done from the position of the analyst.

> The analyst's interpretation merely reflects the fact that the unconscious, if it is what I say it is, namely, a play of the signifier, the unconscious has already in its formations—dreams, slips of tongue or pen, jokes or symptoms—*proceeded by interpretation.* The Other is already there in the very opening, however evanescent, of the unconscious. (S XI.118, N 130; tm)

> At the other extreme [of analytical experience], there is interpretation . . . Interpretation at its term points to desire, with which, in a certain sense, it is identical. When all is said and done, desire is interpretation itself. (S XI.161, N 176; tm)

Unconscious desire proceeds by interpretation; interpretation proceeds by unconscious desire. The unconscious is a reader. The reader is therefore, on some level, always an analysand—an analysand who "knows what he means" but whose interpretation can be given *another reading* than what it means. This is what analytic discourse is all about.

> In analytic discourse, you presume the subject of the unconscious to be capable of reading. This is what this whole affair of the unconscious amounts to. Not only do you presume him to be capable of reading, but you presume him to be capable of learning how to read. (S XX.38)

It is because the unconscious is a reader capable of learning—capable, that is, of learning how to read—that psychoanalysis came into being: the very constitution of psychoanalysis is the outcome, in Lacan's eyes, of an unprecedented, prodigious act of reading. This is how Lacan accounts for the very discovery of the unconscious:

> [Freud's] first interest was in hysteria . . . He spent a lot of time listening, and while he was listening, there resulted something paradoxical, a *reading.* It was while listening to hysterics that he *read* that there was an unconscious. That is, something he could only construct, and in which he himself was impli-

cated; he was implicated in it in the sense that, to his great astonishment, he noticed that he could not avoid participating in what the hysteric was telling him, and that he felt affected by it. Naturally, everything in the resulting rules in which he established the practice of psychoanalysis is designed to counteract this consequence, to conduct things in such a way as to avoid being affected.[3]

■ Freud as Reader

Freud's discovery of the unconscious is the outcome of his reading of the hysterical discourse of his patients, of his being capable of reading in the hysterical discourse of the Other his own unconscious. The discovery of the unconscious is therefore Freud's discovery, within the discourse of the other, of what was actively reading within himself: his discovery, or his reading, of what was reading—in what was being read. Freud's discovery, for Lacan, thus consists not—as it is conventionally understood—of the revelation of a new *meaning* (the unconscious) but of the practical discovery of a new *way of reading*.

In what ways is this unprecedented Freudian act of reading, this inaugural emergence of analytic reading, revolutionary?

(1) Even though Freud's insight springs from a discovery of *what is reading* (his own unconscious) in *what is being read* (the discourse of the hysteric), even though the reading hinges on the reader's own involvement in the subject matter (his "implication" in the symptom observed), the reading is by no means introspective. What Freud reads in the hysteric is not his own resemblance but, rather, his own difference from himself: the reading necessarily passes through the Other, and in the Other, reads not identity (other or same), but difference and self-difference.

(2) Dialogue is not an accident, a contingency of the reading, but its structuring condition of possibility. The reading is revolutionary in that it is essentially, constitutively dialogic. It is grounded in a division; it cannot be synthesized, summed up in a monologue.

(3) "It was while listening to the hysterics that [Freud] read that there was an unconscious. That is, something he could only construct." The unconscious is not, in effect, "discovered"; it is *con-*

structed: it is not a given to be observed, a substance out there that has finally come under the microscope; it is a theoretical construction. The reading is, in other words, of such a nature that it cannot be direct, intuitive; it is constitutively mediated by a hypothesis; it necessitates a theory. But the reading is not theory: it is practice, a practical procedure, partially blind to what it does but which proves to be efficient. The theoretical construction of the unconscious is what, after the fact, is constructed to account for the efficiency of the practice. But the practice, the partially unconscious analytic reading practice, always inescapably precedes the theory. There is a constitutive belatedness of the theory over the practice, the theory always trying to catch up with what it was that the practice, or the reading, was really doing. This belated repetition of the theoretical construction can, however, only partially and asymptotically recover the *primal scene* of analytic reading.

In the perspective of this Lacanian conception of the absolute primacy of Freud's analytic *reading practice* and its precedence over his theory, we might say that Freud's theory of the unconscious is indeed itself nothing other than Freud's constant effort to adjust his own modes of thinking to the availability of his own exemplary lesson of reading.

■ After Freud

Given this grasp of what we may now call Freud's primal scene of reading, Lacan's own analytic theory and practice—his theoretical and practical lesson of reading—turns on this crucial analytic question: What does it mean to be a reader? The question, asked in constant reference to Freud's practice, to Freud's text accounting for his practice, and to Lacan's own analytic practice, comprises three more questions:

What was Freud in effect *doing* as a reader (as a reader of his patients, of the symptom, of his dreams, of literary texts, of his own practice, of his own theoretical constructions)?

What does it mean to be a reader *of* Freud?

What does it mean to be a reader *after* Freud?

These three questions are themselves not so much formulated theoretically as they are pragmatically thought out in each Lacanian reading. This is what I will attempt to show in exploring here in general Lacan's own practice as a reader, and in focusing in particular on two specific Lacanian interpretations: his exemplary and groundbreaking reading of the ways in which psychoanalysis is at stake in a text by Poe (Chapter 2) and his original rereading of the psychoanalytic specimen story of Oedipus (Chapter 5).

CHAPTER TWO ■

The Poe-etic Effect:
A Literary Case History ■

The Psychoanalytical Approaches:
Krutch, Bonaparte, Lacan ■

The Poe-etic Analytical ■

The Case of Poe:
Applications / Implications
of Psychoanalysis

■ Lacan's first collection of published essays, the *Ecrits*, opens with a chapter entitled "The Seminar on *The Purloined Letter*." This so-called "Seminar" is the written account of a year-long course devoted to the exploration of a short literary text, one of Edgar Allan Poe's *Extraordinary Tales*, "The Purloined Letter." The Seminar was offered to trainees in psychoanalysis. Why did Lacan choose to devote a whole year of teaching to this tale? What is the significance of the strategic decision to place this "Seminar" at the opening of the *Ecrits*, as a key work in Lacan's endeavor?

I will approach these questions indirectly, by meditating first on the "case of Poe" in the literary investigations of psychology and psychoanalysis before Lacan. I will then attempt to analyze both the difference that Lacan has made in the psychoanalytical approach to reading and the way in which the lesson Lacan derived from Poe is a lesson in psychoanalysis.

To account for poetry in psychoanalytical terms has traditionally meant to analyze poetry as a symptom of a particular poet. I would here like to reverse this approach, and to analyze a particular poet as a symptom of poetry.

Perhaps no poet has been so highly acclaimed and, at the same time, so violently disclaimed as Edgar Allan Poe. One of the most controversial figures on the American literary scene, "perhaps the most thoroughly misunderstood of all American writers,"[1] "a stumbling block for the judicial critic,"[2] no other poet in the history of criticism has engendered so much disagreement and so many critical contradictions. It is my contention that this critical disagreement is itself symptomatic of a *poetic effect,* and that the critical contradictions to which Poe's poetry has given rise are themselves indirectly significant of the nature of poetry.

■ The Poe-etic Effect: A Literary Case History

No other poet has been so often referred to as a "genius," in a sort of common consensus shared even by his detractors. Joseph Wood Krutch, whose study tends to belittle Poe's stature and to disparage the value of his artistic achievement, nevertheless entitles his monograph *Edgar Allan Poe: A Study in Genius.*[3] So do many other critics, who acknowledge and assert Poe's "genius" in the very titles of their essays.[4] "It happens to us but few times in our lives," writes Thomas Wentworth Higginson, "to come consciously into the presence of that extraordinary miracle we call genius. Among the many literary persons whom I have happened to meet . . . there are not half a dozen who have left an irresistible sense of this rare quality; and among these few, Poe."[5] The English poet Swinburne speaks of "the special quality of [Poe's] strong and delicate genius"; the French poet Mallarmé describes his translations of Poe as "a monument to the genius who . . . exercised his influence in our country"; and the American poet James Russell Lowell, one of Poe's harshest critics, who, in his notorious versified verdict, judged Poe's poetry to include "two fifths sheer fudge," nonetheless asserts, "Mr. Poe has that indescribable something which men have agreed to call *genius* . . . Let talent writhe and contort itself as it may, it has no such magnetism. Larger of bone and sinew it may be, but the wings are wanting."[6]

However suspicious and unromantic the critical reader might wish to be with respect to "that indescribable something which men have agreed to call genius," it is clear that Poe's poetry produces what might be called a *genius effect:* the impression of some undefinable but compelling force to which the reader is subjected. To describe "this power, *which is felt,*"[7] as one reader puts it,

Lowell speaks of "magnetism"; other critics speak of "magic." "Poe," writes Bernard Shaw, "constantly and inevitably produced magic where his greatest contemporaries produced only beauty."[8] T. S. Eliot quite reluctantly agrees: "Poe had, to an exceptional degree, the feeling for the incantatory element in poetry, of that which may, in the most nearly literal sense, be called 'the magic of verse.' "[9]

Poe's "magic" is thus ascribed to the ingenuity of his versification, to his exceptional technical virtuosity. And yet the word *magic,* "in the most nearly literal sense," means much more than just the intellectual acknowledgment of an outstanding technical skill; it connotes the effective action of something that exceeds both the understanding and the control of the person who is subjected to it; it connotes a force to which the reader has no choice but to submit. "No one could tell us what it is," writes Lowell, still in reference to Poe's genius, "and yet there is none who is not inevitably aware of . . . its power" (p. 11). "Poe," said Shaw, "inevitably produced magic." Something about Poe's poetry is experienced as inevitable, unavoidable (and not just as irresistible). What is more, once this poetry is read, its inevitability is there to stay; it becomes lastingly inevitable: "it will stick to the memory of every one who reads it," writes P. Pendleton Cooke (p. 23). And Eliot: "Poe is the author of a few . . . short poems . . . which do somehow stick in the memory" (pp. 207–208).

This is why Poe's poetry can be defined, and indeed has been, as a poetry of influence par excellence, in the sense emphasized by Harold Bloom: "to inflow," or to have power over another. The case of Poe in literary history could in fact be accounted for as an extreme and complex case of "the anxiety of influence," of the anxiety unwittingly provoked by the "influence" irresistibly emanating from this poetry. What is unique, however, about Poe's influence, as about the magic of his verse, is the extent to which its action is unaccountably insidious, exceeding the control, the will, and the awareness of those who are subjected to it. Eliot writes:

> Poe's influence is . . . puzzling. In France the influence of his poetry and of his poetic theories has been immense. In England and America it seems almost negligible . . . And yet

one cannot be sure that one's own writing has *not* been influenced by Poe. (p. 205; original italics)

Studying Poe's influence on Baudelaire, Mallarmé, and Valéry, Eliot goes on to comment:

Here are three literary generations, representing almost exactly a century of French poetry. Of course, these are poets very different from each other . . . But I think we can trace the development and descent of one particular theory of the nature of poetry through these three poets and it is a theory which takes its origin in the theory . . . of Edgar Poe. And the impression we get of the influence of Poe is the more impressive, because of the fact that Mallarmé, and Valéry in turn, did not merely derive from Poe through Baudelaire: each of them subjected himself to that influence directly, and has left convincing evidence of the value which he attached to the theory and practice of Poe himself. (p. 206; original italics)

Curiously enough, while Poe's worldwide importance and effective influence is beyond question, critics nonetheless continue to protest and to proclaim, as loudly as they can, that Poe is unimportant, that Poe is *not* a major poet. Taxing Poe with "vulgarity," Aldous Huxley argues:

Was Edgar Allan Poe a major poet? It would surely never occur to any English-speaking critic to say so. And yet, in France, from 1850 till the present time, the best poets of each generation—yes, and the best critics, too; for, like most excellent poets, Baudelaire, Mallarmé, Paul Valéry are also admirable critics—have gone out of their way to praise him. . . . We who are speakers of English . . . , we can only say, with all due respect, that Baudelaire, Mallarmé, and Valéry were wrong and that Poe is not one of our major poets. (*Recognition*, p. 160)

Poe's detractors seem to be unaware, however, of the paradox that underlies their enterprise: it is by no means clear why anyone should take the trouble to write—at length—about a writer of no importance. Poe's most systematic denouncer, Ivor Winters, thus writes:

The menace lies not, primarily, in his impressionistic admir-
ers among literary people of whom he still has some, even in
England and in America, where a familiarity with his language
ought to render his crudity obvious, for these individuals in
the main do not make themselves permanently very effective:
it lies rather in the impressive body of scholarship . . . When
a writer is supported by a sufficient body of such scholarship,
a very little philosophical elucidation will suffice to establish
him in the scholarly world as a writer whose greatness is self-
evident. (*Recognition*, p. 177)

The irony here is that, in writing his attack on Poe, what the
attacker is in fact doing is adding still another study to the bulk
of "the impressive body of scholarship" in which, in his own terms,
"the menace lies"; so that, paradoxically enough, through Winters'
study, the menace—that is, the possibility of taking Poe's "greatness as a writer" as "self-evident"—will indeed increase. I shall
argue that, regardless of the value-judgment it may pass on Poe,
this impressive bulk of Poe scholarship, the very quantity of the
critical literature to which Poe's poetry has given rise, is itself an
indication of its effective poetic power, of the strength with which
it drives the reader to an *action*, compels him to a *reading act*. The
elaborate written denials of Poe's value, the loud and lengthy negations of his importance, are therefore very like psychoanalytical
negations. It is clear that if Poe's text in effect were unimportant,
it would not seem so important to proclaim, argue, and prove that
he is unimportant. The fact that it so much *matters* to proclaim
that Poe *does not matter* is but evidence of the extent to which
Poe's poetry is, in effect, a poetry that matters.

Poe might thus be said to have a *literary case history*, most
revealing in that it incarnates, in its controversial forms, the paradoxical nature of a strong poetic effect: the very poetry that, more
than any other, is experienced as *irresistible* has also proved to be,
in literary history, the poetry most *resisted*, the one that, more than
any other, has provoked resistances.

This apparent contradiction, which makes of Poe's poetry a
unique case in literary history, clearly partakes of the paradoxical
nature of an *analytical effect*. The enigma it presents us with is the
enigma of the analytical par excellence, as stated by Poe himself,

whose amazing intuitions of the nature of what he calls "analysis" are strikingly similar to the later findings of psychoanalysis: "The mental features discoursed of as the analytical are, in themselves, but little susceptible of analysis. We appreciate them only in their effects."[10]

Because of the very nature of its strong effects, of the reading-acts that it provokes, Poe's text (and not just Poe's biography of his personal neurosis) is clearly an analytical case in the history of literary criticism, a case that suggests something crucial to understand in psychoanalytic terms. It is therefore not surprising that Poe has been repeatedly singled out for psychoanalytical research, has persistently attracted the attention of psychoanalytic critics.

■ The Psychoanalytical Approaches

The best-known and most influential psychoanalytic studies of Poe are the 1926 study by Joseph Wood Krutch and the 1933 study by Marie Bonaparte, *Edgar Poe: Etude psychanalytique.*[11] Through a brief summary of the psychoanalytic issues raised by these two works, I will attempt to analyze the methodological presuppositions guiding their approaches (their "application" of psychoanalysis), in order to compare them later to Lacan's strikingly different approach in his methodologically unprecedented "Seminar on *The Purloined Letter*," published in 1966.[12]

Joseph Wood Krutch: Ideological Psychology, or the Approach of Normative Evaluation

For Krutch, Poe's text is nothing other than an accurate transcription of a severe neurosis, a neurosis whose importance and significance for "healthy" people is admittedly unclear. Poe's "position as the first of the great neurotics has never been questioned," writes Krutch ambiguously. And less ambiguously, in reply to some admiring French definitions of that position: "Poe 'first inaugurated the poetic conscience' only if there is no true poetry except the poetry of morbid sensibility." Since Poe's works, according to Krutch, "bear no conceivable relation . . . to the life of any people, and it is impossible to account for them on the basis of any social or intellectual tendencies or as the expression of the spirit of any age" (p. 210), the only possible approach is a biographical one, and "any true understanding" of the work is contingent upon a diagnosis of Poe's nervous malady. Krutch thus diagnoses in Poe a pathological condition of sexual impotence, the result of a fixation on his mother, and explains Poe's literary drive as a desire to compensate for, on the one hand, the loss of social position of which his foster father had deprived him, through the acquisition of literary fame and, on the other hand, his incapacity to have normal sexual relations, through the creation of a fictional world of horror and destruction where he found refuge. Poe's fascination with logic would thus be merely an attempt to prove himself rational when he felt he was going insane; and his critical theory merely an attempt to justify his peculiar artistic practice.

The obvious limitations of such a psychoanalytic approach were very sharply and accurately pointed out by Edmund Wilson in his essay "Poe at Home and Abroad." Krutch, argues Wilson, seriously misunderstands and undervalues Poe's writings, in

> complacently caricaturing them—as the modern school of social psychological biography, of which Mr. Krutch is a typical representative, seems inevitably to tend to caricature the personalities of its subjects. We are nowadays being edified by the spectacle of some of the principal ornaments of the human race exhibited exclusively in terms of their most ridiculous manias, their most disquieting neurosis, and their most humiliating failures. (*Recognition,* p. 144)

It is, in other words, the reductionist, stereotypical simplification under which Krutch subsumes the complexities of Poe's art and life that renders this approach inadequate:

> Mr. Krutch quotes with disapproval the statement of President Hadley of Yale, in explaining the refusal of the Hall of Fame to accept Poe among its immortals: "Poe wrote like a drunkard and a man who is not accustomed to pay his debts"; and yet Mr. Krutch himself . . . is almost as unperceptive when he tells us, in effect, that Poe wrote like a dispossessed Southern gentleman and a man with a fixation on his mother. (p. 145)

Subscribing to Wilson's criticism, I would like to indicate briefly some further limitations in this type of psychoanalytic approach to literature. Krutch himself, in fact, points out some of the limits of his method in his conclusion:

> We have, then, traced Poe's art to an abnormal condition of
> the nerves and his critical ideas to a rationalized defense of
> the limitations of his own taste . . . The question whether or
> not the case of Poe represents an exaggerated example of the
> process by which all creation is performed is at best an open
> question. The extent to which all imaginative works are the
> result of the unfulfilled desires which spring from either idio-
> syncratic or universally human maladjustments to life is only
> beginning to be investigated, and with it is linked the related
> question of the extent to which all critical principles are at
> bottom the systematized and rationalized expression of in-
> stinctive tastes which are conditioned by causes often un-
> known to those whom they affect. The problem of finding an
> answer to these questions . . . is the one distinctly new problem
> which the critic of today is called upon to consider. He must,
> in a word, endeavor to find the relationship which exists be-
> tween psychology and aesthetics. (pp. 234–35)

This, indeed, is the real question, the real challenge that Poe as
poet (and not as psychotic) presents to the psychoanalytic critic.
But this is precisely the question that is never dealt with in Krutch's
study. Krutch discards the question by saying that "the present
state of knowledge is not such as to enable" us to give any answers.
This remark, however, presupposes that the realm of aesthetics, of
literature and art, might not itself contain some knowledge about,
precisely, "the relationship between psychology and aesthetics"; it
presupposes knowledge as a given, external to the literary object
and imported into it, and not as a result of a reading-process, that
is, of the critic's work upon and with the literary text. It presupposes, furthermore, that a critic's task is not to question but to
answer, and that a question that cannot be answered, can also
therefore not be asked; that to raise a question, to articulate its
thinking power, is not itself a fruitful step that takes some work,
some doing, into which the critic could perhaps be guided by the
text.

Thus, in claiming that he has traced "Poe's art to an abnormal
condition of the nerves," and that Poe's "criticism falls short of
psychological truth," Krutch believes that his own work is opposed
to Poe's as health is opposed to sickness, as normality is opposed

to abnormality, as truth is opposed to delusion. But this ideologically determined, clear-cut opposition between health and sickness
is precisely one that Freud's discovery fundamentally unsettles,
deconstructs. In tracing Poe's "critical ideas to a rationalized defense of the limitations of his own taste," Krutch is unsuspicious
of the fact that his own critical ideas about Poe could equally be
so traced; that his doctrine, were it true, could equally apply to
his own critical enterprise; that if psychoanalysis indeed puts rationality as such in question, it also by the same token puts itself
in question.

Krutch, in other words, reduces not just Poe but analysis itself
into an ideologically biased and psychologically opinionated caricature, missing totally (as is most often the case with "Freudian"
critics) the radicality of Freud's psychoanalytic insights: their self-
critical potential, their power to return upon themselves and to
unseat the critic from any guaranteed, authoritative stance of truth.
Krutch's approach does not, then, make sophisticated use of psychoanalytic insights, nor does it address the crucial question of the
relationship between psychology and aesthetics, nor does it see that
the crux of this question is not so much in the interrogation of
whether or not all artists are necessarily pathological, but of what
it is that makes of art—not of the artist—an object of *desire* for
the public; of what it is that makes for art's effect, for the compelling power of Poe's poetry over its readers. The question of what
makes poetry lies, indeed, not so much in what it was that made
Poe write, but in what it is that makes us read him[13] and that
ceaselessly drives so many people to write about him.

Marie Bonaparte: The Approach of Clinical Diagnosis

In contrast to Krutch's claim that Poe's works are only meaningful
as the expression of morbidity, bearing "no conceivable relation . . . to the life of any people," Marie Bonaparte, although in
turn treating Poe's works as nothing other than the recreations of
his neuroses, tries to address the question of Poe's power over his
readers through her didactic explanation of the relevancy, on the
contrary, of Poe's pathology to "normal" people: the pathological
tendencies to which Poe's text gives expression are an exaggerated
version of drives and instincts universally human, which normal
people have simply repressed more successfully in their childhood.

What fascinates readers in Poe's texts is precisely the unthinkable and unacknowledged but strongly felt community of these human sexual drives.

If Marie Bonaparte, unlike Krutch, thus treats Poe with human sympathy, suspending the traditional puritan condemnation and refraining from passing judgment on his "sickness," she nonetheless, like Krutch, sets out primarily to diagnose that sickness and trace the poetry to it. Like Krutch, she comes up with a clinical portrait of the artist that, in claiming to account for the poetry, once again verges on caricature:

> If Poe was fundamentally necrophilist, as we saw, Baudelaire is revealed as a declared sadist; the former preferred dead prey or prey mortally wounded . . . ; the latter preferred live prey and killing. . . .
>
> How was it then, that despite these different sex lives, Baudelaire the sadist recognised a brother in the necrophilist Poe? . . .
>
> This particular problem raises that of the general relation of sadism to necrophilia and cannot be resolved except by an excursus into the theory of instincts. (p. 680)

Can poetry thus be clinically diagnosed? In setting out to expose didactically the methods of psychoanalytic interpretation, Bonaparte's pioneering book at the same time exemplifies the very naiveté of competence, the distinctive professional crudity of what has come to be the classical psychoanalytic treatment of literary texts. Eager to point out the resemblances between psychoanalysis and literature, Bonaparte, like most psychoanalytic critics, is totally unaware of the differences between the two: unaware of the fact that the differences are as important and as significant for understanding the meeting-ground as are the resemblances, and that those differences also have to be accounted for if poetry is to be understood in its own right. Bonaparte, paradoxically enough but in a manner symptomatic of the whole tradition of applied psychoanalysis, thus remains blind to the very specificity of the object of her research.

It is not surprising that this blind nondifferentiation or confusion of the poetic and the psychotic has unsettled sensitive readers, and that various critics have protested against this all too crude equation of poetry with sickness. The protestations, however, most often fall into the same ideological trap as the psychoanalytical studies they oppose: taking for granted the polarity of sickness versus health, of normality versus abnormality, they simply trace Poe's art (in opposition, so they think, to the psychoanalytic claim) to normality as opposed to abnormality, to sanity as opposed to insanity, to the history of ideas rather than that of sexual drives, to a conscious project as opposed to an unconscious one. Camille Mauclair insists upon the fact that Poe's texts are "constructed objectively by a will absolutely in control of itself," and that genius of that kind is "always sane."[14] For Allen Tate,

> The actual emphases Poe gives the perversions are richer in philosophical implication than his psychoanalytic critics have been prepared to see . . . Poe's symbols refer to a known tradition of thought, an intelligible order, apart from what he was as a man, and are not merely the index to a compulsive neurosis . . . the symbols . . . point towards a larger philosophical dimension. (*Recognition*, p. 239)

For Floyd Stovall, the psychoanalytic studies "are not literary critiques at all, but clinical studies of a supposed psychopathic personality":

> I believe the critic should look within the poem or tale for its meaning, and that he should not, in any case, suspect the betrayal of the author's unconscious self until he has understood all that his conscious self has contributed. To affirm that a work of imagination is only a report of the unconscious is to degrade the creative artist to the level of an amanuensis.
> I am convinced that all of Poe's poems were composed with conscious art. (p. 183) . . .
> "The Raven," and with certain necessary individual differences every other poem Poe wrote, was the product of conscious effort by a healthy and alert intelligence. (p. 186)

It is obvious that this conception of the mutual exclusiveness, of the clear-cut opposition between conscious art and the unconscious, is itself naive and oversimplified. Nonetheless, Stovall's critique of applied psychoanalysis is relevant to the extent that the psychoanalytic explanation, in pointing exclusively to the author's unconscious sexual fantasies, indeed does not account for Poe's outstanding conscious art, for his poetic mastery and his technical and structural self-control. As do its opponents, so does applied psychoanalysis itself fail precisely to account for the dynamic interaction between the unconscious and the conscious elements of art.

If the thrust of the discourse of applied psychoanalysis is, in tracing poetry to a clinical reality, to reduce the poetic to a "cause" outside itself, the crucial limitation of this process of reduction is that the cause, while it may be necessary, is by no means a sufficient one. "Modern psychiatry," judiciously writes David Galloway, "may greatly aid the critic of literature, but . . . it cannot thus far explain why other men, suffering from deprivations or fears or obsessions similar to Poe's, failed to demonstrate his particular creative talent. Though no doubt Marie Bonaparte was correct in seeing Poe's own art as a defense against madness, we must be wary of identifying the necessity for this defense, in terms of Poe's own life, with the success of this defense, which can only be measured in his art."[15]

That the discourse of applied psychoanalysis is limited precisely in that it does not account for Poe's poetic genius is in fact the crucial point made by Freud himself in his prefatory note to Marie Bonaparte's study:

> In this book my friend and pupil, Marie Bonaparte, has shown the light of psychoanalysis on the life and work of a great writer with pathologic trends.
>
> Thanks to her interpretative effort, we now realize how many of the characteristics of Poe's works were conditioned by his personality, and can see how that personality derived from intense emotional fixations and painful infantile experiences. *Investigations such as this do not claim to explain creative genius,* but they do reveal the factors which awake it and the sort of subject matter it is destined to choose.

No doubt, Freud's remarkable superiority over most of his disciples—including Marie Bonaparte—proceeds from his acute awareness of the very limitations of his method, an awareness that in his followers seems most often not to exist.

I would like here to raise a question that has, amazingly enough, never been asked as a serious question: Is there a way around Freud's perspicacious reservation, warning us that studies like those of Bonaparte "do not claim to explain creative genius"? Is there, in other words, a way—a different way—in which psychoanalysis *can* help us to account for poetic genius? Is there an alternative to applied psychoanalysis?—an alternative that would be capable of touching, in a psychoanalytic manner, upon the very specificity of what constitutes the poetic?

Lacan: The Approach of Textual Problematization

"The Purloined Letter," as is well known, is the story of the double theft of a compromising letter, originally sent to the queen. Surprised by the unexpected entrance of the king, the queen leaves the letter on the table in full view of any visitor, where it is least likely to appear suspicious and therefore to attract the king's attention. Enter the Minister D who, observing the queen's anxiety and the play of glances between her and the unsuspicious king, analyzes the situation, figures out, recognizing the addressor's handwriting, what the letter is about, and steals it—by substituting for it another letter he takes from his pocket—under the very eyes of the challenged queen, who can do nothing to prevent the theft without provoking the king's suspicions. The queen then asks the prefect of police to search the minister's apartment and person for the letter. The prefect uses every conceivable secret-police technique to search every conceivable hiding place on the minister's premises, but to no avail.

Having exhausted his resources, the prefect consults Auguste Dupin, the famous "analyst," as Poe calls him (i.e., an amateur detective who excels in solving problems by means of deductive logic), to whom he tells the whole story. (It is, in fact, from this narration of the prefect of police to Dupin and in turn reported by the first-person narrator, Dupin's friend, who is also present, that we, the readers, learn the story.)

On a second encounter, Dupin, to the great surprise of the prefect and of the narrator, produces the purloined letter out of his drawer and hands it to the prefect in return for a large amount of money. The prefect leaves, and Dupin explains to the narrator how he found the letter: he deduced that the minister, knowing that his premises would be thoroughly combed by the police, had concluded that the best principle of concealment would be to leave the letter in the open, in full view; the letter would not be discovered precisely because it would be too self-evident. On this assumption, Dupin called on the minister in his apartment and, glancing around, soon located the letter carelessly hanging from the mantelpiece in a card rack. A little later, a disturbance in the street provoked by a man in Dupin's employ drew the minister to the window, at which moment Dupin quickly replaced the letter with a facsimile.

What Lacan is concerned with at this point of his research is the psychoanalytic problematics of the "repetition compulsion,"[16] as elaborated in Freud's speculative *Beyond the Pleasure Principle*. The thrust of Lacan's endeavor, with respect to Poe, is thus to point out the way in which the story's plot, its sequence of events (as, for Freud, the sequence of events in a life-story), is contingent on, overdetermined by, a principle of repetition that governs it and inadvertently structures its dramatic and ironic impact. "There are two scenes," remarks Lacan, "the first of which we shall straightway designate the primal scene . . . since the second may be considered its repetition in the very sense we are considering today" (p. 41). The primal scene takes place in the queen's boudoir: it is the theft of the letter from the queen by the minister; the second scene—its repetition—is the theft of the letter from the minister by Dupin.

What constitutes repetition for Lacan, however, is not the mere thematic resemblance of the double theft, but the whole structural situation in which the repeated theft takes place: in each case, the theft is the outcome of an intersubjective relationship between three terms; in the first scene, the three participants are the king, the queen, and the minister; in the second, the three participants are the police, the minister, and Dupin. In much the same way as Dupin takes the place of the minister in the first scene (the place of the letter's robber), the minister in the second scene takes the place of the queen in the first (the dispossessed possessor of the letter); whereas the police, for whom the letter remains invisible, take the place formerly occupied by the king. The two scenes thus mirror each other, in that they dramatize the repeated exchange of "three glances, borne by three subjects, incarnated each time by different characters." What is repeated, in other words, is not a psychological act committed as a function of the individual psychology of a character, but three functional *positions in a structure* which, determining three different viewpoints, embody three different relations to the act of seeing—of seeing, specifically, the purloined letter.

The first is a glance that sees nothing: the King and the Police.

The second, a glance which sees that the first sees nothing and deludes itself as to the secrecy of what it hides: the Queen, then the Minister.

The third sees that the first two glances leave what should be hidden exposed to whomever would seize it: the Minister, and finally Dupin. (p. 44)

I have devised the following diagram as an attempt to schematize Lacan's analysis and to make explicit the synchronic, structural perceptions he proposes of the temporal, diachronic unfolding of the drama.

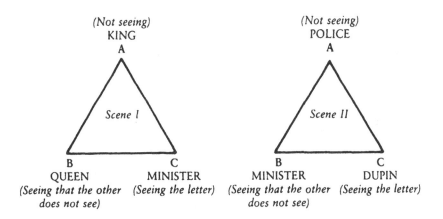

Although Lacan does not elaborate upon the possible ramifications of this structure, the diagram is open to a number of terminological translations, reinterpreting it in the light of Freudian and Lacanian concepts. Here are two such possible translations:

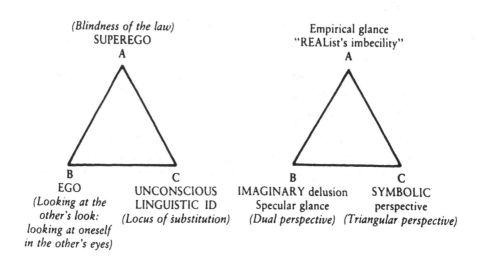

"What interests us today," insists Lacan,

> is the manner in which the subjects relay each other in their displacement during the intersubjective repetition.
>
> We shall see that their displacement is determined by the place which a pure signifier—the purloined letter—comes to occupy in their trio. And that is what will confirm for us its status as repetition automatism. (p. 45)

The purloined letter, in other words, becomes itself—through its insistence in the structure—a symbol or a signifier of the unconscious, to the extent that it is destined "to signify the annulment of what it signifies"—the necessity of its own repression, of the repression of its message: "It is not only the meaning but the text of the message which it would be dangerous to place in circulation" (p. 56). But in much the same way as the repressed *returns* in the *symptom*, which is its repetitive symbolic substitute, the purloined letter ceaselessly returns in the tale—as a signifier of the repressed—through its repetitive displacements and replacements. "This is indeed what happens in the repetition compulsion," says Lacan (p.

60). Unconscious desire, once repressed, survives in displaced symbolic media that govern the subject's life and actions without his ever being aware of their meaning or of the repetitive pattern they structure:

> If what Freud discovered and rediscovers with a perpetually increasing sense of shock has a meaning, it is that the displacement of the signifier determines the subjects in their acts, in their destiny, in their refusals, in their blindnesses, in their end and in their fate, their innate gifts and social acquisitions notwithstanding, without regard for character or sex, and that, willingly or not, everything that might be considered the stuff of psychology, kit and caboodle, will follow the path of the signifier. (p. 60)

In what sense, then, does the second scene in Poe's tale, while repeating the first scene, nonetheless differ from it? In the sense, precisely, that the second scene, through the repetition, allows for an understanding, for an *analysis* of the first. This analysis through repetition is to become, in Lacan's ingenious reading, no less than an *allegory of psychoanalysis*. The intervention of Dupin, who restores the letter to the queen, is thus compared to the intervention of the analyst, who rids the patient of the symptom. The analyst's effectiveness, however, does not spring from his intellectual strength but—insists Lacan—from his position in the repetitive structure. By virtue of his occupying the third position—that is, the *locus* of the unconscious of the subject as a place of substitution of letter for letter (of signifier for signifier)—the analyst, through transference, allows at once for a repetition of the trauma and for a symbolic substitution, and thus effects the drama's denouement.

It is instructive to compare Lacan's study of the psychoanalytical repetition compulsion in Poe's text to Marie Bonaparte's study of Poe's repetition compulsion through his text. Although the two analysts study the same author and focus on the same psychoanalytic concept, their approaches are strikingly different. To the extent that Bonaparte's study of Poe has become a classic, a model of applied psychoanalysis, I would like, in pointing out the differences in Lacan's approach, to suggest the way in which those differences at once put in question the traditional approach and offer an alternative to it.

1. *What does a repetition compulsion repeat? Interpretation of difference as opposed to interpretation of identity.* For Marie Bonaparte, what is compulsively repeated through the variety of Poe's texts is the same unconscious fantasy: Poe's sadonecrophiliac desire for his dead mother. For Lacan, what is repeated in the text is not the content of a fantasy but the symbolic displacement of a signifier through the insistence of a signifying chain; repetition is not of *sameness* but of *difference,* not of independent terms or of analogous themes but of a structure of differential interrelationships,[17] in which what *returns* is always *other.* Thus, the triangular structure repeats itself only through the difference of the characters who successively come to occupy the three positions; its structural significance is perceived only *through* this difference. Likewise, the significance of the letter is situated in its displacement, that is, in its repetitive movements toward a different place. And the second scene, being, for Lacan, an allegory of analysis, is important not just in that it *repeats* the first scene, but in the way this repetition (like the transferential repetition of a psychoanalytical experience) *makes a difference:* brings about a solution to the problem. Thus, whereas Bonaparte analyzes repetition as the insistence of identity, for Lacan any possible insight into the reality of the unconscious is contingent on a perception of repetition, not as a confirmation of identity, but as the insistence of the indelibility of a difference.

2. *An analysis of the signifier as opposed to an analysis of the signified.* In the light of Lacan's reading of Poe's tale as itself an allegory of the psychoanalytic reading, it might be illuminating to define the difference in approach between Lacan and Bonaparte in terms of the story. If the purloined letter can be said to be a sign of the unconscious, for Bonaparte the analyst's task is to uncover the letter's content, which she believes—as do the police—to be hidden somewhere in the real, in some secret biographical depth. For Lacan, on the other hand, the analyst's task is not to read the letter's hidden referential content, but to situate the superficial indication of its textual movement, to analyze the paradoxically invisible symbolic evidence of its displacement, its structural insistence, in a signifying chain. "There is such a thing," writes Poe, "as being too profound. Truth is not always in a well. In fact, as regards the most important knowledge, I do believe she is invariably superficial."[18] Espousing Poe's insight, Lacan makes the principle of symbolic evidence the guideline for an analysis not of the signified

but of the signifier—for an analysis of the unconscious (the re-pressed) not as hidden but on the contrary as *exposed*—in lan-guage—through a significant (rhetorical) displacement.

This analysis of the signifier, the model of which can be found in Freud's interpretation of dreams, is nonetheless a radical reversal of the traditional expectations involved in the common psychoan-alytical approach to literature and its invariable search for hidden meanings. Indeed, not only is Lacan's reading of "The Purloined Letter" subversive of the traditional model of psychoanalytic read-ing: it is, in general, a type of reading that is methodologically unprecedented in the history of literary criticism. The history of reading has accustomed us to the assumption—usually unques-tioned—that reading is finding meaning, that interpretation can dwell only on the meaningful. Lacan's analysis of the signifier opens up a radically new assumption, an assumption that is an insightful logical and methodological consequence of Freud's discovery: that what *can* be read (and perhaps what *should* be read) is not just meaning but the lack of meaning; that significance lies not just in consciousness but, specifically, in its disruption; that the signifier can be analyzed in its effects without its signified being known; that the lack of meaning—the discontinuity in conscious under-standing—can and should be interpreted as such, without neces-sarily being transformed into meaning. "Let's take a look," writes Lacan:

> We shall find illumination in what at first seems to obscure matters: the fact that the tale leaves us in virtually total ig-norance of the sender, no less than of the contents, of the letter. (p. 57)

> The signifier is not functional. . . . We might even admit that the letter has an entirely different (if no more urgent) meaning for the Queen than the one understood by the Minister. The sequence of events would not be noticeably affected, not even if it were strictly incomprehensible to an uninformed reader. (p. 56)

> But that this is the very effect of the unconscious in the precise sense that we teach that the unconscious means that man is inhabited by the signifier. (p. 66)

Thus, for Lacan, what is analytical par excellence is not (as is the case for Bonaparte) the readable but the unreadable and the effects of the unreadable. What calls for analysis is the insistence of the unreadable in the text.

Poe, of course, had said it all in his comment on the nature of what he too—amazingly enough, before the fact—called "the analytical": "The mental features discoursed of as the analytical are, in themselves, but little susceptible of analysis. We appreciate them only in their effects." But, oddly enough, what Poe himself had said so strikingly about the analytical had itself remained totally unanalyzed, indeed unnoticed, by psychoanalytic scholars before Lacan, perhaps because it, too, according to its own analytical logic, had been "a little too self-evident" to be perceived.

3. *A textual as opposed to a biographical approach.* The analysis of the signifier implies a theory of textuality for which Poe's biography, or his so-called sickness, or his hypothetical personal psychoanalysis, become irrelevant. The presupposition—governing enterprises like that of Marie Bonaparte—that poetry can be interpreted only as autobiography is obviously limiting and limited. Lacan's textual analysis for the first time offers a psychoanalytical alternative to the previously unquestioned and thus seemingly exclusive biographical approach.

4. *The analyst/author relation: a subversion of the master/slave pattern and of the doctor/patient opposition.* Let us remember how many readers were unsettled by the humiliating and sometimes condescending psychoanalytic emphasis on Poe's "sickness," as well as by an explanation equating the poetic with the psychotic. There seemed to be no doubt in the minds of psychoanalytic readers that if the reading situation could be assimilated to the psychoanalytic situation, the poet was to be equated with the sick patient, with the analysand on the couch. Lacan's analysis, however, subverts not only this clinical status of the poet, but along with it the "bedside" security of the interpreter. If Lacan is not concerned with Poe's sickness, he is quite concerned nonetheless with the figure of the poet in the tale, and with the hypotheses made about his specific competence and incompetence. Both the minister and Dupin are said to be poets, and it is their *poetic* reasoning that the prefect fails to understand and that thus enables both to outsmart the police. "D——, I presume, is not altogether a fool,"

comments Dupin early in the story, to which the prefect of police replies:

> "Not altogether a fool . . . but then he's a poet, which I take to be only one remove from a fool."
> "True," said Dupin, after a long and thoughtful whiff from his meerschaum, "although I have been guilty of certain doggerel myself." (p. 334)

A question Lacan does not address could be raised by emphasizing still another point that would normally tend to pass unnoticed, since, once again, it is both so explicit and so ostentatiously insignificant: Why does Dupin say that he too is *guilty* of poetry? In what way does the status of the poet involve guilt? In what sense can we understand the guilt of poetry?

Dupin, then, draws our attention to the fact that both he and the minister are poets, a qualification to which the prefect is condescending. Later, when Dupin explains to the narrator the prefect's defeat, he again insists upon the prefect's blindness to a logic or to a "principle of concealment" which has to do with poets and thus (it might be assumed) is specifically poetic:

> This functionary has been thoroughly mystified; and the remote source of his defeat lies in the supposition that the Minister is a fool, because he has acquired renown as a poet. All fools are poets; this the Prefect feels; and he is merely guilty of a *non distributio medii* in thence inferring that all poets are fools. (pp. 341–324)

In Baudelaire's translation of Poe's tale into French, the word *fool* is rendered, in its strong, archaic sense, as *fou*, "mad." Here, then, is Lacan's paraphrase of this passage in the story:

> After which, a moment of derision [on Dupin's part] at the Prefect's error in deducing that because the Minister is a poet, he is not far from being mad, an error, it is argued, which would consist . . . simply in a false distribution of the middle term, since it is far from following from the fact that all madmen are poets.
> Yes indeed. But we ourselves are left in the dark as to the poet's superiority in the art of concealment. (p. 52)

Both this passage in the story and this comment by Lacan seem to be marginal, incidental. Yet the hypothetical *relationship between poetry and madness* is significantly relevant to the case of Poe and to the other psychoanalytical approaches we have been considering. Could it not be said that the error of Marie Bonaparte (who, like the prefect, engages in a search for hidden meaning) lies precisely in the fact that, like the prefect once again, she simplistically equates the poetic with the psychotic, and so, blinded by what she takes to be the poetic *incompetence,* fails to see or understand the specificity of poetic *competence?* Many psychoanalytic investigations diagnosing the poet's sickness and looking for his poetic secret in his person (as do the prefect's men) are indeed very like police investigations; and like the police in Poe's story, they fail to find the letter, fail to see the textuality of the text.

Lacan, of course, does not say all this—this is not what is at stake in his analysis. All he does is open up still another question where we believed we had come into possession of some sort of answer:

> Yes indeed. But we ourselves are left in the dark as to the poet's superiority in the art of concealment.

This seemingly lateral question, asked in passing and left unanswered, suggests, however, the possibility of a whole different focus or perspective of interpretation in the story. If "The Purloined Letter" is specifically the story of "the poet's superiority in the art of concealment," then it is not just an allegory of psychoanalysis but also, at the same time, an allegory of poetic writing. And Lacan is himself a poet to the extent that a thought about poetry is what is superiorly concealed in his Seminar.

In Lacan's interpretation, however, the poet's superiority can only be understood as the structural superiority of the third position with respect to the letter: the minister in the first scene, Dupin in the second, both poets. But the third position is also—this is the main point of Lacan's analysis—the position of the analyst. It follows that, in Lacan's approach, the status of the poet is no longer that of the sick patient but, if anything, that of the analyst. If the poet is still the object of the accusation of being a fool, his folly— if it does exist (which remains an open question)—would at the same time be the folly of the analyst. The clear-cut opposition between madness and health, or between doctor and patient, is unsettled by the odd functioning of the purloined letter of the unconscious, which no one can possess or master. "There is no metalanguage," says Lacan: there is no language in which interpretation can itself escape the effects of the unconscious; the interpreter is not more immune than the poet to unconscious delusions and errors.

5. *Implication, as opposed to application, of psychoanalytic theory.* Lacan's approach no longer falls into the category of what has been called "applied psychoanalysis," since the concept of application implies a relation of exteriority between the applied science and the field it is supposed, unilaterally, to inform. Since, in Lacan's analysis, Poe's text serves to reinterpret Freud just as Freud's text serves to interpret Poe; since psychoanalytic theory and the literary text mutually inform—and displace—each other; since the very position of the interpreter—of the analyst—turns out to be not outside but inside the text, there is no longer a clear-cut opposition or a well-defined border between literature and psychoanalysis: psychoanalysis can be intraliterary just as much as literature is intrapsychoanalytic. The methodological stake is no longer that of the *application* of psychoanalysis *to* literature but, rather, of their *interimplication in* each other.

If I have dealt at length with Lacan's innovative contribution and with the different methodological example of his approach, it is not so much to set this example up as a new model for imitation, but rather to indicate the way in which it suggestively invites us to go beyond itself (as it takes Freud beyond itself), the way in which it opens up a whole new range of as yet untried possibilities for the enterprise of reading. Lacan's importance in my eyes does not, in other words, lie specifically in any new dogma his "school" may propose, but in his outstanding demonstration that *there is more than one way* to implicate psychoanalysis in literature; that *how to* implicate psychoanalysis in literature is itself a question for interpretation, a challenge to the ingenuity and insight of the interpreter, and not a *given* that can be taken in any way for granted; that what is of analytical relevance in a text is not necessarily and not exclusively "the unconscious of the poet," let alone his sickness or his problems in life; that to situate in a text the analytical as such—to situate the object of analysis or the textual point of its implication—is not necessarily to recognize a *known*, to find an answer, but also, and perhaps more challengingly, to locate an *unknown,* to find a question.

■ The Poe-etic Analytical

Let us now return to the crucial question we left in suspension earlier, after having raised it by reversing Freud's reservation concerning Marie Bonaparte's type of research: Can psychoanalysis give us an insight into the specificity of the poetic? We can now supplement this question with a second one: where can we situate the analytical with respect to Poe's poetry?

The answers to these questions might be sought in two directions. (1) In a direct reading of a poetic text by Poe, trying to locate in the poem itself a signifier of poeticity and to analyze its functioning and its effects; to analyze, in other words, how poetry as such works through signifiers (to the extent that signifiers, as opposed to meanings, are always signifiers of the unconscious); (2) in an analytically informed reading of literary history itself, since its treatment of Poe obviously constitutes a literary *case history.* Such a reading has never, to my knowledge, been undertaken with respect to any writer: never has literary history itself been viewed as an analytical object, as a subject for a psychoanalytic interpretation.[19] And yet it is overwhelmingly obvious, in a case like Poe's, that the discourse of literary history itself points to some unconscious determinations that structure it but of which it is not aware. What is the unconscious of literary history? Can the question of *the guilt of poetry* be relevant to that unconscious? Could literary history be in any way considered a repetitive unconscious *transference* of the guilt of poetry?

Literary history, or more precisely the critical discourse surrounding Poe, is indeed one of the most visible ("self-evident") effects of Poe's poetic signifier, of his text. Now, how can the question of the peculiar effect of Poe be dealt with analytically? My suggestion is: by locating what seems to be unreadable or incomprehensible in this effect; by situating the most prominent discrepancies or discontinuities in the overall critical discourse concerning Poe, the most puzzling critical contradictions, and by trying to interpret those contradictions as symptomatic of the unsettling specificity of the Poe-etic effect, as well as of the contingence of such an effect on the unconscious.

According to its readers' contradictory testimonies, Poe's poetry, let it be recalled, seemed to be at once the most *irresistible* and the most *resisted* poetry in literary history. Poe is felt to be at once the most unequaled master of conscious art *and* the most tortuous unconscious case, as such doomed to remain "the perennial victim of the *idée fixe,* and of amateur psychoanalysis."[20] Poetry, I would thus argue, is precisely the effect of a deadly struggle between consciousness and the unconscious; it has to do with resistance and with what can neither be resisted nor escaped. Poe is a symptom of poetry to the extent that poetry is both what most resists a psychoanalytical interpretation and what most depends on psychoanalytical effects.

But this, paradoxically enough, is what poetry and psychoanalysis have in common. They both exist only insofar as they resist our reading. When caught in the act, both are always already, once again, purloined.

CHAPTER THREE ∎

What Difference Does Psychoanalysis Make? or The Originality of Freud

■ "Conservatism," writes Charles Sanders Peirce, "in the sense of a dread of consequences, is altogether out of place in science— which has on the contrary always been forwarded by radicals and radicalism, in the sense of the eagerness to carry consequences to their extremes."[1] Simply put, the originality of Lacan lies in his radical understanding of the radicality of Freud's discovery, and in his eagerness to carry the consequences of this discovery to their logical limits. In so doing, Lacan assesses and thinks out not just the significance of psychoanalysis but, specifically, the significance of the difference that it makes, of the difference it has introduced into Western culture. Lacan's originality, in other words, lies in his uncompromising inquiry into the originality of psychoanalysis.

Lacan himself refers to his own originality only to disclaim it: "What I have just said," he writes in the inaugural Rome Discourse—the first important exposition of his theoretical innovations—"what I have just said has so little originality, even in its verve, that there appears in it not a single metaphor that Freud's works do not repeat with the frequency of a leitmotif" (E260, N51). And on another inaugural occasion, the first issue of his periodical *Scilicet*, Lacan repeats: "The originality we are allowed is limited to the scrap of enthusiasm we have adopted . . . concerning what Freud was able to name" (*Scilicet* 1, 6). By his own definition Lacan's originality is, paradoxically enough, nothing other than the originality of repetition: the originality of a *return* . . . to Freud.

How can a return be original? This is, among other things, what Lacan would make us understand. And indeed one of the consequences of Lacan's originality is, precisely, a displacement of the very concept of originality.

Lacan's well-known inaugural call for the return to Freud is itself an operation—and a notion—far more complex, far more original than the simple gesture it customarily is understood to be: it is not simply a historical return to the authentic origin of a doctrine, nor even a return to Freud's original text as opposed, on the one hand, to its dogmatic, oversimplified interpretations and, on the other, to its inaccurate translations. It is a return to Freud *untranslated* as a symptom of the essential untranslatability of his subject matter. Freud himself, indeed, often compared the unconscious to a foreign language and defined repression as a constitutive "failure of translation." It is thus no coincidence that Lacan's return to Freud is dramatized as a literal, concrete return to a foreign language, to something that defies translation: it is a return whose function, paradoxically, is not so much to render Freud familiar as to renew contact with his strangeness: a return to a Freud constitutively foreign—even to himself; a return to Freud's struggle with the radical impossibility of translation; a return to the unconscious—both *in* Freud's text and *of* Freud's text—not as a domesticated, reassuring answer but as an irreducibly uncanny question.[2]

Since what returns in the Lacanian "return" is precisely what is unassimilable in Freud, the return to Freud is not unlike the return of the repressed: it partakes itself of the dimension of a symptom, which Lacan defines as "the return of truth . . . in the discrepancy of knowledge." Like the symptom, the return to Freud involves "a mnemonic element of a privileged anterior situation which is repeated so as to articulate a current situation" (E 447). Freud's originality is indeed not unlike the originality of a trauma, which takes on meaning only through the deferred action of a return. Freud's discovery of the unconscious can thus itself be looked at as a sort of primal scene, a cultural trauma, whose meaning—or originality in cultural history—comes to light only through Lacan's significantly transferential, symptomatic repetition.

■ Analytic Dialogue, or the Two-Way Return

What the return to Freud constitutes is a sort of *analytic* dialogue between Lacan and Freud. Freud is returned to as the Other, who returns to Lacan his own message in a reversed, displaced form.

> The Other is, therefore, the locus in which is constituted the I who speaks together with the one who hears, that which is said by the one being already the reply . . . But *in return* this locus also extends as far into the subject as the laws of speech, that is to say, well beyond the discourse that takes its catch-words from the ego. (E 431, N 141; tm)

> All these indications cross-check, overlap one another and these overlappings assure us, in our turn, that we are rejoining Freud—without being able to know for sure whether it is from this source in Freud that our Ariadne's thread has come to us, because, of course, we had read it before formulating our theory of the signifier, but without always understanding it, at the moment. It is no doubt through the particular necessities of our expertise that we have set at the heart of the structure of the unconscious the causal gap, but the fact that we now find an enigmatic, unexplained indication of it in Freud's text is for us a sign that we are progressing in the way of *his* certainty. For *the subject of certainty is divided here.* (S xi.46–47, N 46; tm)

This passage illustrates the way in which the return to Freud is not a one-way path to an already constituted truth, but a *two-way return* that is itself constitutive of truth. This means that truth is correlative with the discrepancy that conditions and necessitates the return. The subject of certainty is radically divided. The dynamic structure is irreducible, irreducibly untotalizable.

The two-way return is thus structured like an analytic dialogue between what Lacan—with significant ambiguity—entitles, "The Freudian Unconscious and Ours" (title of chapter 2, S xi.21, N 17). "The Freudian Unconscious" can designate either Freud's concept of the unconscious or Freud's own unconscious. The same ambiguity applies to "Ours." The dialogue between the two is neither simply conceptual (a dialogue between the two conceptions of the unconscious, Freud's and ours) nor simply transferential (a dialogue between Lacan's and Freud's actual unconscious), but a complex interaction between concept and transference, theory and symptom—through the active mediation of their signifying language; an interaction in which Lacan at times comes to occupy, in Freud's text, the eccentric place of Freud's unconscious, and Freud, from a different vantage point, occupies the place of Lacan's unconscious. The dialogue is analytical in that it is not equal to the sum of its parts; the knowledge for which the analytic dialogue is a vehicle is not reducible to the sum total of the knowledge of each of its two subjects. In Lacan's terminology, it is not a dialogue between two egos, it is not reducible to a dual relationship between *two* terms, but is constituted by a third term that is the meeting point in language between Lacan's and Freud's unconscious: a linguistic, signifying meeting place that is the locus of Lacan's insight but that Lacan does not master. Lacan's originality is thus the originality of a return in that it is irreducibly dialogic.

■ The Originality of Psychoanalysis

That originality *as such* is radically dialogic—necessarily passing through the Other—is, precisely, what psychoanalysis has taught Lacan: this is also, in Lacan's conception, the very gist of the originality of psychoanalysis.

The specific question of the originality of psychoanalysis is indeed the original focus—I would even say, the original desire—of Lacan's interrogation. Instead of asking, in the classical tradition of Freud's commentators, what is the content of the knowledge Freud has bequeathed us, Lacan asks: What is the difference this knowledge makes? What specifically distinguishes this new knowledge from former knowledge? What is the consequence of this new knowledge with respect to former knowledge, what does it do to former knowledge? And still more radically: What is the process, the original procedure, by which Freud arrives at whatever knowledge he bequeathes us? What is the specificity, or the originality, of what Freud has instituted, without even assuming in advance that it necessarily consists of knowledge? To put it in Lacan's own emphatic, passionate terms: "What is this something, which analysis teaches us which is specific, proper to it [*qui lui soit propre*], or the most proper, truly proper?" (E 440).

Psychoanalysis, in Lacan's view, consists of three interrelated elements, each having an originality of its own:

Psychoanalysis, first and foremost, is a *praxis* (a practical treatment of a patient, the concrete process of an analysis).

Psychoanalysis is a *method*, a technique put to use in the praxis.

Psychoanalysis is a *theory*.

In Lacan's conception, the originality of the praxis lies in its "intersubjective play through which truth enters into the real" (E 438). The originality of the praxis is, in other words, structural: "The praxis that we call psychoanalysis is constituted by a structure" (E 793, N 292). The original structure is precisely the structure of psychoanalytic dialogue—different from the binary structure of the conventional notion of dialogue—a structure Lacan will for the first time attempt to systematize. "Whereas the condition of analysis is such," says Lacan, "that the true work it executes remains by its nature hidden, this is not the case with the structure of analysis, which one can formalize in a manner entirely accessible to the scientific community" (E 438).

As for the theory of psychoanalysis, its originality, for Lacan, consists not so much in Freud's discovery of the unconscious—intuited before him by the poets—as in Freud's unprecedented discovery of the fact that *the unconscious speaks:* that the unconscious has a logic or a signifying structure, that it is structured like a language. This is what constitutes the radicality of the Freudian unconscious, which is not simply *opposed* to consciousness but speaks as something other *from within* the speech of consciousness, which it subverts. The unconscious is thenceforth no longer—as it has traditionally been conceived—the simple outside of the conscious, but rather a division, *Spaltung*, cleft within consciousness itself; the unconscious is no longer the difference between consciousness and the unconscious, but rather the inherent, irreducible difference between consciousness and itself. The unconscious, therefore, is the radical castration of the mastery of consciousness, which turns out to be forever incomplete, illusory, and self-deceptive.

> The Freudian unconscious has nothing to do with the so-called forms of the unconscious that preceded it . . . and which still surround it today . . . forms of the unconscious which will tell nobody anything that he did not already know, and which

simply designate *the non-conscious,* the more or less conscious, etc. . . .

Freud's unconscious is not at all the romantic unconscious of imaginative creation. It is not the locus of the divinities of the night . . . Psychoanalysis is introducing something other . . .

To all these forms of the unconscious, ever more or less linked to some obscure will regarded as primordial, to something pre-conscious, what Freud opposes is the revelation that at the level of the unconscious there is something at all points homologous with what occurs at the level of the subject—*this thing speaks* [ça parle] and functions in a way quite as elaborate as at the level of the conscious, which thus loses what seemed to be its privilege. (S XI.26–27, N 24)

As for the psychoanalytic method, on the other hand, its originality lies in its manipulation of the signifier, that is, in its manipulation of unconscious symbolic effects through its exclusive use of language. The fact that Freud decided not to use the apparently more convenient tool of hypnosis is crucial to the understanding of the meaning of his method. "For if the originality of the analytic method is constituted by the means it deprives itself of, it is because the means to which it confines itself are enough to constitute a domain whose limits define the relativity of its operations" (E 257, N 49; tm).

■ The First Analysis: The Inaugural Procedure

Behind the psychoanalytic method, what emerges, then, is Freud's inaugural procedure. This constitutive procedure—to which Lacan devotes singular attention—is indeed what is most original in the joint constitution of psychoanalytic practice, theory, and method: it is the very principle of originality which has brought about the difference named psychoanalysis. Lacan writes:

I insist on the fact that Freud advanced in an investigation which is not marked by the same style as other scientific investigations. His domain is that of the truth of the subject. The investigation of truth is not entirely reducible to the objective, and even objectifying, investigation of the common scientific method. What is at stake is the realization of the truth of the subject, a dimension specific to psychoanalysis and whose originality has to be detached even from the very notion of reality . . .

Freud was engaged in the investigation of a truth which concerned him totally in his very person, therefore also in his presence to the patient, in his activity . . . as a therapist.

Certainly, analysis as a science is always a science of the particular. The realization of an analysis is always a singular case, even though those singular cases lend themselves to some generality. But the psychoanalytic experience with Freud represents singularity pushed to its extreme, since Freud was in the process of constructing and of verifying analysis itself. We cannot erase this fact, that this was the first time an analysis had taken place. The method was, no doubt, deduced from this first analysis, but it is only for others that it becomes a method. Freud, for his part, was not applying a method. If we neglect the unique, inaugural character of his procedure, we shall be committing a serious error.

Analysis is an experience of the particular. The truly original experience of this particularity takes on here an even more singular value. If we do not emphasize the difference that exists between this *first time* and everything that followed—we who are pursuing, not so much the truth as the access-routes to that truth—we will never be able to grasp the meaning [of Freud's work]." (S I.29)

What does the "first time," the inaugural access route to the truth, consist of? It consists, as we have seen, of the negative procedure by which Freud chooses to forego hypnosis; it consists, therefore, in Freud's exclusive concentration on the discourse of the hysteric. It is indeed the discourse of the hysteric which will give birth to nothing less than the new science of psychoanalysis. How?

For there lies the meaning, which is not emphasized enough, of the distance which Freud takes with respect to hypnoid states, a distance from which Freud proceeds, when the question is that of explaining even merely the phenomena of hysteria. This is the stypefying fact: Freud prefers the discourse of the hysteric. (E 795, N 294; tm)

This indicates that Freud places his certainty, his *Gewiss-heit,* only in the constellation of the signifiers as they result from the recounting, the commentary, the association, even if they are later retracted. Everything provides signifying material, which is what he depends on to establish his own *Ge-wissheit*—for I stress the fact that analytical experience begins only with his way of proceeding, with his method. (S XI.44–45, N 44; tm)

How, then, does the method arise out of the radicality of this inaugural way of proceeding, out of Freud's elimination of all knowledge or information other than that furnished by the discourse of the hysteric? As we have seen earlier,[3] Freud's discovery of the unconscious is the outcome of his being capable of reading in the hysterical discourse of the Other his own unconscious. The discovery of the unconscious was Freud's discovery, within the discourse of the other, of what was actively reading within himself.

■ A New Mode of Reflexivity

What Lacan thus brings to light is the fact that what Freud's "inaugural step"—his constitutive procedure—inaugurates and later institutes is a new and unprecedented *mode of reflexivity*—of the process through which something turns back upon itself: a new mode of reflexivity that necessarily incorporates a passage through the Other, not as a reflection of the self but as a radical difference from the self, a radical difference to which, paradoxically, the very movement of reflexivity is addressed; a reflexivity whose self-reference, whose process of turning back upon itself, is not based on symmetry but on asymmetry: asymmetry between the self departed from and the self returned to; asymmetry between the turn and the return; a reflexivity, therefore, which, passing through the Other, returns to itself without quite being able to rejoin itself; a reflexivity which is thus untotalizable, that is, irreducibly dialogic, and in which what is returned to the self from the Other is, paradoxically, the ignorance or the forgetfulness of its own message; a reflexivity, therefore, which is a new mode of cognition or information gathering whereby ignorance itself becomes structurally informative, in an asymmetrically reflexive dialogue in which the interlocutors — through language—inform each other of what they do not know.

What Lacan also points out for the first time is the way in which this new Freudian mode of reflexivity *differs* from the traditional humanistic mode of reflexivity, from the classical psychological and philosophical epistemology of *self-reflection*. Self-reflection, the traditional fundamental principle of consciousness and of conscious thought, is what Lacan traces back to "the mirror stage," to the symmetrical dual structure of the Imaginary. Self-reflection is always a mirror reflection, that is, the illusory functioning of symmetrical reflexivity, of reasoning by the illusory principle of symmetry between self and self as well as between self and other; a symmetry that subsumes all difference within a delusion of a unified and homogenous individual identity. But the new Freudian mode of reflexivity precisely shifts, displaces, and unsettles the very boundaries between self and other, subverting by the same token the symmetry that founds their dichotomy, their clear-cut opposition to each other.

By shifting and undercutting the clear-cut polarities between subject and object, self and other, inside and outside, analyst and analysand, consciousness and the unconscious, the new Freudian reflexivity substitutes for all traditional binary, symmetrical conceptual oppositions—that is, substitutes for the very foundations of Western metaphysics—a new mode of interfering heterogeneity. This new reflexive mode—instituted by Freud's way of listening to the discourse of the hysteric and which Lacan will call "the in-mixture of the subjects" (E 415)—divides the subjects differently, in such a way that they are neither entirely distinguished, separate from each other, nor, correlatively, entirely totalizable but, rather, interfering from within and in one another.

■ A New Model of Scientificity

If, however, the originality of Freud's procedure consists in its being singularly reflexive and reflexively singular, how can Freud be sure that his reflexive method touches upon the real, or at the very least is in touch with a structural truth? Freud's method of verification, in Lacan's analysis, is again reflexive: it consists in the way in which the different reflexive gestures, the different dialogically reflexive interpretations, meet one another, find themselves—by an insistent chance—structurally cross-checked to and cross-checked by one another:

And there is only one method of knowing that one is there, namely, to map the network. And how is a network mapped? It is through the fact that one returns, one comes back, one keeps coming across the same path, it always overlaps and cross-checks itself in the same way [ça se recoupe toujours de la même façon]; and in this seventh chapter of *The Interpretation of Dreams* there is no other confirmation for one's *Gewissheit*, one's certainty, than this—"Speak of chance, gentlemen, if you like. In my experience I have observed nothing arbitrary in this field, for it always meets up with itself, it cross-checks itself in such a way that it escapes chance." (S xi.45, N 45; tm)

As you saw with the notion of intersection or overlapping [recoupement], the function of return, *Wiederkehr*, is essential. It is not only *Wiederkehr* in the sense of that which has been repressed—the very constitution of the field of the unconscious is based on the *Wiederkehr*. It is there that Freud bases his certainty. But it is quite obvious that it is not from there that it comes to him. It comes to him from the fact that in the process he recognizes the law of his own desire. He would not have been able to advance in this wager of certainty if he had not been guided in it, as his writings show, by his *self-analysis* . . . Freud advances, sustained by a certain relation to his desire, and by what constitutes his act, namely, the constitution of psychoanalysis. (S xi.48, N 47–48; tm)

The self-analysis—another structural, dynamic reflexivity—thus comes to confirm the reflexivity of Freud's observations of his patients. In that the reflexive operation of the self-analysis cross-checks Freud's dialogically reflexive interpretation of his patients, or his reflexive interpretation of the Oedipus myth, it becomes a reflexivity to the second degree, that is, a reflexivity itself engaged in an analytic dialogue with the otheness of another reflexivity. And it is through this function of return—of the two-way return between dialogic reflexivities—that these extreme operations of singularity and particularity can be generalized into laws from which psychoanalysis emerges not just as practice and as method but as theory.

Thus it is Freud who, from his first methodological step concerning the hysteric to the constitution of his theory, understands and puts in action the originality of the new mode of return. Paradoxically enough, it was Freud himself who was the first to inaugurate, investigate, and redefine the implications of a *return to Freud*. But is is Lacan who makes us see how the complex originality of Freud's return to Freud constitutes a radically new model of scientificity.

■ The Symptoms of a Science

"What we ought to emphasize here," writes Lacan, "is our claim to be opening up the path of the scientific position, insofar as we are analyzing the way in which that position is already implicated at the very root of the psychoanalytical discovery":

> The reformulation of the subject, which is inaugural here, should be linked to the reformulation produced by the very principle of science—science itself entailing a certain postponement with respect to those ambiguous questions that can be called questions of truth. (E 234)

In modern science, indeed, the object of observation is no longer considered a given. It is constructed, by means of a hypothesis without which the observation—the process of confirmation or invalidation of the hypothesis—would not take place. The physicist is himself part of the data, the experimenter part of the laboratory. The observer is a fundamental structural, desiring, formative part of the observed. Modern science, in other words, includes the symptom of the observer in the observed. But this is precisely, in Lacan's conception, the gist of Freud's radical operation:

> We are only bringing this up in order to put in relief the *leap* involved in Freud's operation.
>
> What is distinctive about Freud's operation is that it clearly articulates the status of the symptom with the status of its own discourse, for it constitutes precisely the very *operation proper to the symptom,* in both senses of the word. (E 234)

That is, I believe, Lacan's most crucial, most far-reaching, insight: to have analyzed Freud's constitutive operation as itself proceeding from the symptom that is its object, to have analyzed psychoanalysis as itself proceeding from Freud's transference, but to have done so not—in the narrow-minded manner of psychologizing critics—so as to discard the theory, to invalidate or reduce the operation—but, on the contrary, so as to account for its new principle of fecundity and for its revolutionary type of scientific rigor.

■ Freud's Copernican Revolution

Freud himself compared the radicality of his discovery to the scientific revolution brought about by Copernicus, and Lacan likes to return to that comparison. Freud writes:

> In the early stages of his researches, man believed at first that his dwelling-place, the earth, was the stationary center of the universe, with the sun, moon and planets circling round it. In this he was naively following the dictates of his sense-perceptions, for he felt no movement of the earth, and wherever he had an unimpeded view he found himself in the center of a circle that enclosed the external world. The central position of the earth, moreover, was a token to him of the dominating part played by it in the universe and appeared to fit in very well with his inclination to regard himself as lord of the world.
>
> The destruction of this narcissistic illusion is associated in our minds with the name and work of Copernicus. (SE 18.139–140)

Just as Copernicus discovers that it is not the sun that revolves around the earth but the earth that revolves around the sun, so Freud displaces the center of the human world from consciousness to the unconscious. "Human megalomania," in Freud's terms, thus suffers another "wounding blow" from the psychoanalytical discovery that "the ego . . . is not even master of its own house, but must content itself with scanty information of what is going on unconsciously in its mind" (SE 17.285). Freud himself thus defines his own originality as subversive: subversive of the principle of consciousness as a center and, along with it, of man's narcissistic centrality to himself.

It is interesting to see how Lacan's originality redefines Freud's originality, through a *return* to the very same Copernican reference. For Lacan emphasizes not so much the scientific consequence of the change of center as the scientific *process* of decentering, that is, the new mode of reflexivity: "But Freud's discovery was to demonstrate that this verifying process authentically attains the subject only by decentering him from consciousness-of-self" (E 292, N 80). For Lacan, then, Freud—like Copernicus—stands not so much as the discoverer of a new center but as the discoverer of a new mode of reflexivity for which the celestial revolution[4]—the revolving movement of the planets—becomes itself an ingenious metaphor, something like a geometric figure. "The revolution is no less important," says Lacan, "for concerning only the 'celestial revolutions' " (E 757, N 295). But again Lacan emphasizes the crucial fact that the Freudian celestial revolution—or revolving reflexivity—is radically tied up with language:

> It was in fact the so-called Copernican revolution to which Freud himself compared his discovery, emphasizing that it was once again a question of the place man assigns to himself at the center of a universe.
>
> It is not a question of knowing whether I speak of myself in a way that conforms to what I am, but rather of knowing whether I am the same as that of which I speak.
>
> Is the place that I occupy as the subject of a signifier con-centric or eccentric, in relation to the place I occupy as subject of the signified? (E 516–517, N 165)

What difference does Lacan's emphasis on language make for the understanding of the significance of the privileged metaphor of Copernican revolution?

Freud concentrates on the revolutionized status of the center and of centrality; Lacan on the revolutionized conception of the very moment of revolving. Freud therefore emphasizes the revolution-ized *observed*—the resulting revolutionized image of the human mind; Lacan brings out the implication of the revolutionized sci-entific *status of the observer*. In Freud's emphasis, if the Copernican revolution replaces one center with another, displaces the centrality from earth to sun, one could still conceive of the planets as sepa-rable, self-contained spatial entities: one could still think of the two centers—the mistaken and the real one—as distinct from each other. In Lacan's explicitly and crucially linguistic model of reflex-ivity, there are no longer distinct centers but only contradictory gravitational pulls. The two pseudo-centers—"the subject of the signifier" (of the utterance) and "the subject of the signified" (of the statement)—even though they are radically different from each other, are no longer entirely distinct and cannot be separated from each other: each can also be the Other, is "inmixed" with the Other.

Lacan thus brings out the originality of Freud's Copernican revolution by radicalizing the ambiguity between the two centers. In so doing he pursues Freud's discovery, curiously enough, in the same way that Kepler, Copernicus' disciple, discovered in his turn, on the basis of his predecessor's investigations, that the revolving movement of the planets is in fact not *circular* but *elliptical,* that is, revolving not around one but around two so-called foci.

■ Elliptical Necessities

I am not absolutely sure that Lacan—as a subject of the signified— actually made all this entirely explicit to himself. But as a subject of the signifier, his insightful style is uncannily in touch with Freud's radical reflexivity—with Freud's Copernican revolution—in both senses of the word. Lacan thus writes:

> The linguistically suggestive use of Copernicus' name has more hidden resources than touch specifically on what has just slipped from my pen as the relation to the true, namely, the emergence of the ellipse as being not unworthy of the locus from which the so-called higher truths take their name. The revolution is no less important for concerning only the "celestial revolutions." (E 797, N 295)

There are two signifying centers in this quotation, two key words on which Lacan is playing: the word *ellipse* and the word *revolution.* Each of these words has in turn two discrete semantic centers. Lacan is playing, first of all, on the double meaning of the French word *ellipse,* which designates at once the noncircular, non-uni-centered spatial itinerary of the planets—the *geometric figure* of their movement of revolving and, on the other hand, the *rhetorical figure* of speech named *ellipsis,* by which parts of meaning (parts of the signified) are eclipsed, omitted. Lacan, elliptically, does not articulate either the discrepancy or the relation between those two meanings, but he offers them to the reader's ear as resonances. We can understand that it is because the subject is *decentered,* is pulled so to speak bifocally in two different gravitational directions, that his speech becomes necessarily elliptical—that parts of it drop into the unconscious—the unconscious being, in Lacan's conception, precisely that part of the subject's discourse which, although it regulates the subject's actions, is nonetheless not at his disposal: that part which cannot be spoken, constituted as it is by a "failure of translation."

Thus, in Lacan's linguistic play on the metaphor of the Copernican revolution, the key word of the revolution—*ellipse*—itself elliptically revolves around two distinct foci, illustrating, in a concrete linguistic manner, the radical ambiguity of centrality, the radically elliptical reflexivity that is indeed what the Copernican-Freudian revolution is all about.

Lacan's style is thus not mere word play, nor is it just—as is often said—a stylistic imitation of the rhetoric of the unconscious: it is a perpetual reenactment of Freud's elliptical reflexivity, of Freud's Copernican revolution in both senses of the word.

For the word *revolution* itself (in the last passage quoted from Lacan: "the revolution is no less important for concerning only the 'celestial revolutions' ") also plays the double game of turning back upon itself, being repeated twice with two different signifieds, having in its turn two ambiguous semantic centers, the one meaning revolution as subversion, an epistemological break or scientific leap, and the other meaning—as in "the celestial revolutions"—almost the exact opposite: the very movement of turning round, of revolving, of endlessly returning to the same place, of repeating. It is the word *revolution* itself that finally returns upon itself but, in returning to itself, returns to a difference from itself, becomes in fact semantically contradictory with itself, that is, subverts itself: subverts itself as a univocal and totalizable meaning. In Lacan's terms, it becomes a signifier.

What Lacan implicitly suggests is that Freud's discovery of the radically dialogic mode of elliptical reflexivity revolutionizes, among other things, the very notion of revolution or, to put it differently, the very notion of *originality*. Originality is what comes as a surprise: a surprise not only to the others, but also to the self. True originality, in other words, is precisely the way in which a reflexive movement, in returning to and upon itself, in effect *subverts itself*— finds something other than what it had expected, what it had set out to seek; the way in which the answer is bound in effect to displace the question; the way in which what is revolving, what returns to itself, radically displaces the very point of observation. This, at least, was the originality of Freud's discovery, and of Lacan's rediscovery—of Freud.

CHAPTER FOUR ■

Psychoanalysis and Education: Teaching Terminable and Interminable

■ As a question in which practice, rather than a theory, is staked, the unconscious, in Lacan's view, is grounded not so much in an ontological as in an ethical experience:

> The status of the unconscious, which, as I have suggested, is so fragile on the ontic plane, is ethical: in his thirst for truth, Freud says, *Whatever may happen, it is imperative to go there.*
> (S xi, N 33)

How to go there? Is "how to go there" teachable? In what way is the question of teaching related to what Lacan significantly calls *the ethics of psychoanalysis?*

Asked by Meno, "Can you tell me, Socrates, if virtue can be taught?" Socrates replies: "I am so far from knowing whether virtue can be taught or not that I do not even have any knowledge of what virtue itself is." "Yes, Socrates," insists Meno, "but how do you mean that we do not learn, but that what we call learning is recollection? Can you teach me how this is so?" "Meno," says Socrates, "you are a rascal. Here you are asking me to give you my 'teaching,' I who claim that there is no such thing as teaching, only recollection."[1] Socrates, that extraordinary teacher who taught humanity what pedagogy is, and whose name personifies the birth of pedagogics as a science, thus inaugurates his teaching practice, paradoxically enough, by asserting not just his own ignorance but the radical impossibility of teaching.

Another extraordinarily effective pedagogue, another one of humanity's great teachers, Freud, repeats the same conviction that teaching is a fundamentally impossible profession. "None of the applications of psychoanalysis," he writes, "has excited so much interest and aroused so many hopes . . . as its use in the theory and practice of education": "My personal share in this application of psychoanalysis has been very slight. At an early stage I had accepted the *bon mot* which lays it down that there are three impossible professions—educating, healing, governing—and I was already fully occupied with the second of them" (SE 19.273). In a later text—indeed the very last one he wrote—Freud recapitulates this paradoxical conviction that time and experience seem to have only confirmed: "It almost looks as if analysis were the third of those 'impossible' professions in which one can be sure beforehand of achieving unsatisfying results. The other two, which have been known much longer, are education and government" (SE 23.248).

If teaching is impossible, what are we teachers doing? How should we understand—and carry out—our task? And why is it that two of the most effective teachers ever to appear in the intellectual history of mankind regard the task of teaching as impossible? Indeed, is not their enunciation of the impossibility of teaching itself actively engaged in teaching, itself part of the lesson they bequeath us? And, if so, what can be learned from the fact that it is impossible to teach? What can the impossibility of teaching teach us? As much as Socrates, Freud has instituted, among other things, a revolutionary pedagogy. It is precisely in giving us unprecedented insight into the impossibility of teaching that psychoanalysis has opened up unprecedented teaching possibilities, renewing both the questions and the practice of education.

This pedagogical renewal was not, of course, systematically thought out by Freud himself or systematically articulated by any of his followers; nor have its thrust and scope been fully assimilated or fully grasped, let alone utilized in the classroom. One truly different pedagogy that has emerged from what might be called the psychoanalytic lesson is the thoroughly original teaching style of Lacan. If Lacan, as I have argued, exemplifies the most radical effect of the insights of Freud's teaching, perhaps his teaching practice might give us a clue to the newness of the psychoanalytic lesson about lessons, and help us thus to define both the actual and, more

important, the potential contribution of psychoanalysis to pedagogy.

▪ What Is a Critique of Pedagogy?

Lacan's relationship with pedagogy has itself been oversimplified,
misunderstood, reduced. The reason for the usual misinterpretations of both Lacan's and Freud's pedagogical contribution lies in
a misunderstanding of the critical position taken by psychoanalysis
with respect to traditional methods and assumptions of education.
Lacan's well-known critique of what he has pejoratively termed
"academic discourse" (*le discours universitaire*) situates "the radical vice" in "the transmission of knowledge." "A Master of Arts,"
writes Lacan ironically, "as well as other titles, protect the secret
of a substantialized knowledge." Lacan thus blames "the narrow-
minded horizon of pedagogues" for having reduced the strong
notion of teaching to a "functional apprenticeship" (E 445).[2]

Whereas Lacan's pedagogical critique is focused on grown-up
training—on academic education and the ways it handles and structures knowledge—Freud's pedagogical critique is mainly concerned
with children's education and the ways it handles and structures
repression. "Let us make ourselves clear," writes Freud, "as to
what the first task of education is":

> The child must learn to control his instincts. It is impossible
> to give him liberty to carry out all his impulses without re-
> striction . . . Accordingly, education must inhibit, forbid and
> suppress, and this is abundantly seen in all periods of history.
> But we have learnt from analysis that precisely this suppression
> of instincts involves the risk of neurotic illness . . . Thus ed-
> ucation has to find its way between the Scylla of non-inter-
> ference and the Charybdis of frustration . . . An optimum must
> be discovered which will enable education to achieve the most
> and damage the least . . . A moment's reflection tells us that
> hitherto education has fulfilled its task very badly and has
> done children great damage. (SE 22.149)

Thus, in its most massive statements and in its polemical pro-
nouncements, psychoanalysis is first and foremost a critique of
pedagogy. The legacy of this critique, however, has been miscon-

strued and greatly oversimplified, in that the critical stance has been understood—in both Lacan's and Freud's case—as a desire to escape the pedagogical imperative: a desire to do away with pedagogy altogether. "Psychoanalysis," writes Anna Freud, "whenever it has come into contact with pedagogy, has always expressed the wish to limit education. Psychoanalysis has brought before us the quite definite danger arising from education."[3]

The illocutionary force of the psychoanalytic critique of pedagogy has thus been reduced, either to a simple negativity or to a simple positivity of that critique. Those who, in an oversimplification of the Freudian lesson, equate the psychoanalytic critical stance with a simple positivity give positive advice to educators, in an attempt to conceive of more liberal methods for raising children—methods allowing "to each stage in the child's life the right proportion of instinct-gratification and instinct-restriction."[4] Those who, on the other hand, in an oversimplification of the Lacanian lesson, equate the psychoanalytical critical stance with a simple negativity see in psychoanalysis "literally an inverse pedagogy": "the analytic process is in effect a kind of reverse pedagogy, which aims at undoing what has been established by education."[5] In the title of one book on the relation of Freud to pedagogy, Freud is thus defined as "The Anti-Pedagogue."[6] This one-sided negative interpretation fails to see that every true pedagogue is in effect an anti-pedagogue, not just because every pedagogy has historically emerged as a critique of pedagogy (Socrates: "There's a chance, Meno, that we, you as well as me . . . have been inadequately educated, you by Gorgias, I by Prodicus"), but because in one way or another every pedagogy stems from its confrontation with the impossibility of teaching (Socrates: "You see; Meno, that I am not teaching . . . anything, but all I do is question"). The reductive conception of "Freud, the anti-pedagogue" thus fails to see that there is no such thing as an anti-pedagogue: an anti-pedagogue is *the* pedagogue par excellence. Such a conception overlooks, indeed, Freud's own stupendous pedagogical performance and its relevance to his declarations about pedagogy.

The trouble both with the positivistic and the negativistic misinterpretations is that they refer exclusively to Lacan's or Freud's explicit *statements* about pedagogy and thus fail to see the illocutionary force, the didactic function, of the *utterance* as opposed to the mere content of the statement. They fail to see, in other words, the pedagogical situation—the dynamic in which statements function not as simple truths but as performative speech acts. Invariably, all existing psychoanalytically inspired theories of pedagogy fail to address the question of the pedagogical speech act of Freud himself or of Lacan himself: what can be learned about pedagogy not just from their theories (which only fragmentarily and indirectly deal with the issue of education) but from their way of teaching it, from their own practice as teachers, their own pedagogical performance.

Lacan refers explicitly to the psychoanalyst's "mission of teaching" (E 241, N 34; tm) and speaks of his own teaching—the bimonthly seminar he gave for forty years—as a vocation, "a function . . . to which I have truly devoted my entire life" (S XI.7, N 1). Freud addresses the issue of teaching more indirectly, rather by refusing to associate with it:

> But there is one topic which I cannot pass over so easily— not, however, because I understand particularly much about it or have contributed very much to it. Quite the contrary: I have scarcely concerned myself with it at all. I must mention it because it is so exceedingly important, so rich in hopes for the future, perhaps the most important of all the activities of analysis. What I am thinking of is the application of psychoanalysis to education. (SE 22.146)

This statement promotes pedagogy to the rank of "perhaps the most important of all the activities of analysis" only on the basis of Freud's denial of his personal involvement with it. However, this very denial is itself engaged in a dramatic pedagogical performance; it is itself part of an imaginary "lecture," significantly written in the form of an academic public address and of a dialogue with students—a dialogue imaginarily conducted by a man who, in reality terminally ill and having undergone an operation for mouth cancer, is no longer capable of speech:

> My *Introductory Lectures on Psychoanalysis* were delivered . . . in a lecture room of the Vienna Psychiatric Clinic before an audience gathered from all the Faculties of the University . . .

These new lectures, unlike the former ones, have never been delivered. My age had in the meantime absolved me from the obligation of giving expression to my membership in the University (which was in any case a peripheral one) by delivering lectures; and a surgical operation had made speaking in public impossible for me. If, therefore, I once more take my place in the lecture room during the remarks that follow, it is only by an artifice of the imagination; it may help me not to forget to bear the reader in mind as I enter more deeply into my subject . . . Like their predecessors, [these lectures] are addressed to the multitude of educated people to whom we may perhaps attribute a benevolent, even though cautious, interest in the characteristics and discoveries of the young science. This time once again it has been my chief aim to make no sacrifice to an appearance of being simple, complete or rounded-off, not to disguise problems and not to deny the existence of gaps and uncertainties. (SE 22.5–6)

No other such coincidence of fiction and reality, biography and theory, could better dramatize Freud's absolutely fundamental pedagogic gesture. What better image could there be for the pedagogue in spite of himself, the pedagogue in spite of everything—the dying teacher whose imminent death, like that of Socrates, only confirms that he is a born teacher—than this pathetic figure, this living allegory of the speechless speaker, of the teacher's teaching out of—through—the radical impossibility of teaching?

Pedagogy in psychoanalysis is thus not just a theme: it is a rhetoric. It is not just a statement: it is an utterance. It is not just a meaning: it is action; an action that itself may very well at times belie the stated meaning, the didactic thesis, the theoretical assertion. It is essential to become aware of this complexity of the relation of pedagogy and psychoanalysis, in order to begin to think out what the psychoanalytic teaching about teaching might be.

Discussing "The Teaching of Psychoanalysis in Universities," Freud writes: "it will be enough if [the student] learns something about psychoanalysis and something from it" (SE 17.73). To learn something *from* psychoanalysis is a very different thing than to learn something *about* it: it means that psychoanalysis is not a simple object of the teaching, but its subject. In his "Psychoanalysis and Its Teaching," Lacan underlines the same ambiguity, the same dynamic complexity, indicating that the true object of psychoanalysis, the object of his teaching, can only be that mode of learning which institutes psychoanalysis itself as subject—as the purveyor of the act of teaching. "How can what psychoanalysis teaches us be taught?" he asks (E 439).

As myself both a student of psychoanalysis and a teacher, I would here like to suggest that the lesson to be learned about pedagogy from psychoanalysis is less that of "the application of psychoanalysis to pedagogy" than that of the implication of psychoanalysis in pedagogy and of pedagogy in psychoanalysis. Attentive thus both to the pedagogical speech act of Freud and to the teaching practice of Lacan, I would like to address the question of teaching as itself a psychoanalytic question. Reckoning not just with the pedagogical thematics *in* psychoanalysis but with the pedagogical rhetoric *of* psychoanalysis, not just with what psychoanalysis says about teachers but with psychoanalysis itself as teacher, I will attempt to analyze the ways in which—modifying the conception of what learning is and of what teaching is—psychoanalysis has shifted pedagogy by radically displacing our very modes of intelligibility.

■ Analytical Apprenticeship

Freud conceives of the process of a psychoanalytic therapy as a learning process—an apprenticeship whose epistemological validity far exceeds the contingent singularity of the therapeutic situation:

> Psychoanalysis sets out to explain . . . uncanny disorders; it engages in careful and laborious investigations . . . until at length it can speak thus to the ego:
>
> " . . . A part of the activity of your own mind has been withdrawn from your knowledge and from the command of your will . . . you are using one part of your force to fight the other part . . . A great deal more must constantly be going on in your mind than can be known to your consciousness. Come, *let yourself be taught* . . . ! What is in your mind does not coincide with what you are conscious of; whether something is going on in your mind and whether you hear of it, are two

different things. In the ordinary way, I will admit, the intelligence which reaches your consciousness is enough for your
needs; and you may cherish the illusion that you learn of all
the more important things. But in some cases, as in that of an
instinctual conflict... your intelligence service breaks
down... In every case, the news that reaches your consciousness is incomplete and often not to be relied on... Turn your
eyes inward... learn first to know yourself!... "
    It is thus that psychoanalysis has sought to educate the ego.
(SE 17.142–143)

Psychoanalysis is a pedagogical experience. As a process that gives
access to new knowledge previously denied to consciousness, it
affords what might be called a lesson in cognition (and in miscog-
nition), an epistemological instruction.

Psychoanalysis institutes in this way a unique and original mode
of learning: original not only in its procedures but in the fact that
it gives access to information unavailable through any other mode
of learning—unprecedented information, hitherto unlearnable. "We
learnt," writes Freud, "a quantity of things which could not have
been learnt except through analysis" (SE 22.147).

This new mode of investigation and learning has, however, a
very different temporality from the conventional linear—cumula-
tive and progressive—temporality of learning, as it has traditionally
been conceived by pedagogical theory and practice. Proceeding not
through linear progression but through breakthroughs, leaps, discontinuities, regressions, and deferred action, the analytic learning
process puts in question the traditional pedagogical belief in intellectual perfectibility, the progressist view of learning as a simple
one-way road from ignorance to knowledge.

It is in effect the very concept of both ignorance and knowledge—the understanding of what "to know" and "not to know"
may really mean—that psychoanalysis has modified, renewed. And
it is precisely the originality of this renewal which is central to
Lacan's thought, to Lacan's specific way of understanding the cultural, pedagogical and epistemological revolution implied by the
discovery of the unconscious.

■ Knowledge

Western pedagogy can be said to culminate in Hegel's philosophical didacticism. The Hegelian concept of "absolute knowledge"—which for Hegel defines at once the potential aim and the actual end of dialectics, of philosophy—is what pedagogy has always aimed at as its ideal: the exhaustion—through methodical investigation— of all there is to know; the absolute completion—termination— of apprenticeship. Complete and totally appropriated knowledge will become, in all senses of the word, a *mastery*. "In the Hegelian perspective," writes Lacan, "the completed discourse" is "an in- strument of power, the scepter and the property of those who know" (S II.91). "What is at stake in absolute knowledge is the fact that discourse closes back upon itself, that it is entirely in agreement with itself."

But the unconscious, in Lacan's conception, is precisely the dis- covery that human discourse can by definition never be entirely in agreement with itself, entirely identical to its knowledge of itself, since, as the vehicle of unconscious knowledge, it is constitutively the material locus of a signifying difference from itself.

Indeed, the unconscious itself is a kind of *unmeant knowledge* that escapes intentionality and meaning, a knowledge spoken by the language of the subject (spoken, for instance, by his "slips" or by his dreams), but that the subject cannot recognize, assume as his, appropriate; a speaking knowledge nonetheless denied to the speaker's knowledge. In Lacan's own terms, the unconscious is "knowledge that can't tolerate one's knowing that one knows" (Seminar, 19 February 1974, unpublished). "Analysis appears on the scene to announce that there is knowledge that does not know itself, knowledge that is supported by the signifier as such" (S xx.88). "It is from a place that differs from any capture by a subject that a knowledge is surrendered, since that knowledge offers itself only to the subject's slips—to his misprision" (*Scilicet* 38). "The discovery of the unconscious . . . is that the implications of meaning infinitely exceed the signs manipulated by the individual" (S II.150). "As far as signs are concerned, man is always mobilizing many more of them than he knows" (S II.150).

If this is so, there can be no such thing as absolute knowledge: absolute knowledge is knowledge that has exhausted its own ar- ticulation, but articulated knowledge is by definition what cannot

exhaust its own self-knowledge. For knowledge to be spoken, lin-
guistically articulated, it would constitutively have to be supported
by the ignorance carried by language, the ignorance of the *excess
of signs* that of necessity its language—its articulation—"mobi-
lizes." Thus human knowledge is, by definition, that which is untotalizable, that which rules out any possibility of totalizing what
it knows or of eradicating its own ignorance.

The epistemological principle of the irreducibility of ignorance
that stems from the unconscious receives an unexpected confirmation from modern science, to which Lacan is equally attentive
in his attempt to give the theory of the unconscious its contemporary scientific measure. The scientific atotality of knowledge
is acknowledged by modern mathematics, in set theory (Cantor:
"The set of all sets in a universe does not constitute a set"). In contemporary physics, it is the crux of the uncertainty principle of
Heisenberg:

> This is what the Heisenberg principle amounts to. When it is
> possible to locate, to define precisely one of the points of the
> system, it is impossible to formulate the others. When the place
> of electrons is discussed . . . it is no longer possible to know
> anything about . . . their speed. And inversely . . . (S ii.281)

From the striking and instructive coincidence between the revolutionary findings of psychoanalysis and the new theoretical orientation of modern physics, Lacan derives the following
epistemological insight, a pathbreaking pedagogical principle:

> Until further notice, we can say that *the elements do not an-
> swer in the place where they are interrogated.* Or more exactly,
> as soon as they are interrogated somewhere, it is impossible
> to grasp them in their totality. (S ii.281)

■ Ignorance

Ignorance is thus no longer simply opposed to knowledge: it is
itself a radical condition, an integral part of the very structure of
knowledge. But what does ignorance consist of, in this new epistemological and pedagogical conception?

If ignorance is to be equated with the atotality of the unconscious, it can be said to be a kind of forgetting—of forgetfulness:

while learning is obviously remembering and memorizing ("all learning is recollection," says Socrates), ignorance is linked to what is not remembered, what will not be memorized. But what will not be memorized is tied up with repression, with the imperative to forget—the imperative to exclude from consciousness, not to admit to knowledge. Ignorance, in other words, is not a passive state of absence, a simple lack of information: it is an active dynamic of negation, an active refusal of information. Freud writes:

> It is a long superseded idea . . . that the patient suffers from a sort of ignorance, and that if one removes this ignorance by giving him information (about the causal connection of his illness with his life, about his experiences in childhood, and so on) he is bound to recover. The pathological factor is not his ignorance in itself, but the root of this ignorance in his *inner resistances;* it was they who first called this ignorance into being, and they still maintain it now. The task of the treatment lies in combating these resistances. (SE 9.225)

Teaching, like analysis, has to deal not so much with lack of knowledge as with resistances to knowledge. Ignorance, suggests Lacan, is a passion. Inasmuch as traditional pedagogy postulated a desire for knowledge, an analytically informed pedagogy has to reckon with "the passion for ignorance" (S xx.110). Ignorance, in other words is nothing other than a *desire to ignore:* its nature is less cognitive than performative. As in the case of Sophocles' nuanced representation of the ignorance of Oedipus, it is not a simple lack of information but the incapacity—or the refusal—to acknowledge one's own implication in the information.

The new pedagogical lesson of psychoanalysis is not subsumed, however, by the revelation of the dynamic nature, and of the irreducibility, of ignorance. The truly revolutionary insight—the truly revolutionary pedagogy discovered by Freud—consists in showing the ways in which ignorance itself can teach us something, become itself instructive. This is, indeed, the crucial lesson that Lacan learned from Freud:

> It is necessary, says Freud, to interpret the phenomenon of doubt as an integral part of the message. (S 11.155)

> The forgetting of the dream is . . . itself part of the dream. (S 11.154)

The message is not forgotten in just any manner . . . A censorship is an intention. Freud's argumentation properly reverses the burden of the proof—"In these elements that you cite in objection to me, the memory lapses and the various degradations of the dream, I continue to see a meaning, and even an additional meaning. When the phenomenon of forgetting intervenes, it interests me all the more . . . *These negative phenomena, I add them to the interpretation of the meaning. I recognize that they too have the function of a message.* Freud discovers this dimension . . . What interests Freud . . . [is] the message as an interrupted discourse, and which insists. (S II.153)

The pedagogical question crucial to Lacan's own teaching will thus be: Where does it resist? Where does a text (or a signifier in a patient's conduct) precisely make no sense, that is, resist interpretation? Where does what I see and what I read resist my understanding? Where is the ignorance—the resistance to knowledge—located? And what can I learn from the locus of that ignorance? How can I interpret *out of* the dynamic ignorance I analytically encounter, both in others and in myself? How can I turn ignorance into an instrument of teaching?

Teaching is something rather problematic . . . As an American poet has pointed out, no one has ever seen a professor who has fallen short of the task because of ignorance . . .

One always knows enough in order to occupy the minutes during which one exposes oneself in the position of the one who knows . . .

This makes me think that there is no true teaching other than the teaching which succeeds in provoking in those who listen an insistence—this desire to know which can only emerge when they themselves have taken the measure of ignorance as such—of ignorance inasmuch as it is, as such, fertile—in the one who teaches as well. (S II.242)

■ The Use of That Which Cannot Be Exchanged

Teaching, thus, is not the transmission of ready-made knowledge. It is rather the creation of a new condition of knowledge, the creation of an original learning disposition. "What I teach you," says Lacan, "does nothing other than express the condition thanks to which what Freud says is possible" (S 11.368). The lesson, then, does not "teach" Freud: it teaches the condition that makes it possible to learn Freud—the condition that makes possible Freud's teaching. What is this condition?

In anaylsis, what sets in motion the psychoanalytical apprenticeship is the peculiar pedagogical structure of the analytic situation. The analysand speaks to the analyst, whom he endows with the authority of the one who possesses knowledge—knowledge of what is precisely lacking in the analysand's own knowledge. The analyst, however, knows nothing of the sort. His only competence, insists Lacan, lies in "what I would call *textual knowledge,* so as to oppose it to the referential notion which only masks it" (*Scilicet* 21). Textual knowledge—the very stuff the literature teacher is supposed to deal in—is knowledge of the functioning of language, of symbolic structures, of the signifier, knowledge at once derived from—and directed toward—interpretation.

But such knowledge cannot be acquired (or possessed) once and for all: each case, each text, has its own specific, singular symbolic functioning and requires a different interpretation. The analysts, says Lacan, are "those who share this knowledge only at the price, on the condition of their not being able to exchange it" (*Scilicet* 59). Analytic (textual) knowledge cannot be *exchanged,* it has to be *used*—and used in each case differently, according to the singularity of the case, according to the specificity of the text. Textual or analytic knowledge is, in other words, that peculiarly specific knowledge which, unlike any commodity, is subsumed by its *use* value, having no exchange value whatsoever.[7] Analysis thus has no use for ready-made interpretations, for knowledge given in advance. Lacan insists on "the insistence with which Freud recommends to us to approach each new case as if we had never learnt anything from his first interpretations" (*Scilicet* 20). "What the analyst must know," concludes Lacan, "is how to ignore what he knows."

■ Dialogic Learning, or the Analytical Structure of Insight

Each case is thus, for the analyst as well as for the patient, a new apprenticeship. "If it is true that our knowledge comes to the rescue of the patient's ignorance, it is not less true that, for our part, we, too, are plunged in ignorance" (S 1.78). While the analysand is obviously ignorant of his own unconscious, the analyst is doubly ignorant: pedagogically ignorant of his suspended (given) knowledge; actually ignorant of the very knowledge the analysand presumes him to possess of his own (the analysand's) unconscious: knowledge of the very knowledge he—the patient—lacks. In what way does knowledge, then, emerge in and from the analytic situation?

Through the analytic dialogue the analyst, indeed, has first to learn where to situate the ignorance: where his own textual knowledge is *resisted*. It is, however, out of this resistance, out of the patient's active ignorance, out of the patient's speech which says much more than it itself knows, that the analyst will come to *learn* the *patient's own* unconscious *knowledge,* that knowledge which is inaccessible to itself because it cannot tolerate knowing that it knows; and it is the signifiers of this constitutively a-reflexive knowledge coming from the patient that the analyst *returns* to the patient from his different vantage point, from his non-reflexive, asymmetrical position as an Other. Contrary to the traditional pedagogical dynamic, in which the teacher's question is addressed to an answer from the other—from the student—which is totally reflexive, and expected, "the true Other," says Lacan, "is the Other who gives the answer one does not expect" (S 11.288). Coming from the Other, knowledge is, by definition, that which comes as a surprise, that which is constitutively the return of a difference:

TEIRESIAS ... *You* are the land's pollution.

OEDIPUS How shamelessly you started up this taunt! How do you think you will escape?

TEIRESIAS ... I have escaped; the truth is what I cherish and that's my strength.

OEDIPUS And who has taught you truth? Not your profession surely!

TEIRESIAS You have taught me, for you have made me speak against my will.

> OEDIPUS Speak what? Tell me again that I may learn it better.
>
> TEIRESIAS Did you not understand before or would you pro-
> voke me into speaking?
>
> OEDIPUS I did not grasp it, not so to call it known. Say it
> again.
>
> TEIRESIAS I say you are the murderer of the king whose mur-
> derer you seek.[8]

As Teiresias—in order to articulate the truth—must have been *taught* not by his profession but *by* Oedipus, so the analyst precisely must be taught by the analysand's unconscious. It is by structurally occupying the position of the analysand's unconscious, and by thus making himself a *student of the patient's knowledge,* that the analyst becomes the patient's teacher—makes the patient learn what would otherwise remain forever inaccessible to him.

For teaching to be realized, for knowledge to be learned, the position of alterity is therefore indispensable: knowledge is what is already there, but always in the Other. Knowledge, in other words, is not a substance but a structural dynamic; it is not contained by any individual but comes about out of the mutual apprenticeship between two partially unconscious speeches that both say more than they know. Dialogue is thus the radical condition of learning and of knowledge, the analytically constitutive condition through which ignorance becomes structurally informative; knowledge is essentially, irreducibly dialogic. "No knowledge," writes Lacan, "can be supported or transported by one alone" (*Scilicet* 59).

Like the analyst, the teacher cannot in turn be, alone, a master of the knowledge he teaches. Lacan transposes the radicality of analytic dialogue—as a newly understood structure of insight—into the pedagogical situation. This is not simply to say that he encourages "exchange" and calls for students' interventions, as many other teachers do. Much more profoundly and radically, he attempts to learn from the students his own knowledge. It is the following original pedagogical appeal that he can thus address to the audience of his seminar:

> It seems to me I should quite naturally be the point of convergence of the questions that may occur to you.
>
> Let everybody tell me, in his own way, his idea of what I

am driving at. How, for him, is opened up—or closed—or how already he resists, the question as I pose it. (S II.242)

■ The Subject Presumed To Know

This pedagogical approach, which makes no claim to total knowledge, which does not even claim to be in possession of its own knowledge, is of course quite different from the usual pedagogical pose of mastery, different from the image of the self-sufficient, self-possessed proprietor of knowledge. This figure of infallible human authority implicitly likened to a God, both modeled on and guaranteed by divine omniscience, is based on an illusion: the illusion of a consciousness transparent to itself. "It is the case of the unconscious," writes Lacan, "that it abolishes the postulate of the subject presumed to know" (*Scilicet* 46).

Abolishing a postulate, however, does not mean abolishing an illusion: whereas psychoanalysis uncovers the mirage inherent in the function of the subject presumed to know, it also shows the prestige and the affective charge of that mirage to be constitutively irreducible, to be indeed most crucial to the emotional dynamic of all discursive human interactions, of all human relationships founded on sustained interlocution. The psychoanalytical account of the functioning of this dynamic is the most directly palpable, the most explicit lesson psychoanalysis has taught us about teaching.

In a brief and peculiarly introspective essay called "Some Reflections on Schoolboy Psychology," the already aging Freud nostalgically probes into his own schoolboy psychology, the affect of which even time and intellectual achievements have not entirely extinguished. "As little as ten years ago," writes Freud, "you may have had moments at which you suddenly felt quite young again":

> As you walked through the streets of Vienna—already a greybeard and weighed down by all the cares of family life—you might come unexpectedly on some well-preserved, elderly gentleman, and would greet him humbly almost, because you had recognized him as one of your former schoolmasters. But afterwards, you would stop and reflect: 'Was that really he? or only someone deceptively like him? How youthful he looks! And how old you yourself have grown! . . . Can it be possible

that the men who used to stand for us as types of adulthood were so little older than we were?' (SE 13.241)

Commenting on his emotion at meeting an old schoolmaster, Freud goes on to give an analytical account of the emotional dynamic of the pedagogical situation:

It is hard to decide whether what affected us more . . . was our concern with the sciences that we were taught or with . . . our teachers . . . In many of us the path to the sciences led only through our teachers . . .

We courted them and turned our backs on them, we imagined sympathies and antipathies which probably had no existence . . . psychoanalysis has taught us that the individual's emotional attitudes to other people . . . are . . . established at an unexpectedly early age . . . The people to whom [the child] is in this way fixed are his parents . . . His later acquaintances are . . . obliged to take over a kind of emotional heritage; they encounter sympathies and antipathies to the production of which they themselves have contributed little . . .

These men [the teachers] became our substitute fathers. That was why, even though they were still quite young, they struck us as so mature and so unattainably adult. We transferred to them the respect and expectations attaching to the omniscient father of our childhood, and then we began to treat them as we treated our own fathers at home. We confronted them with the ambivalence that we had acquired in our own families and with its help we struggled with them as we had been in the habit of struggling with our fathers. (SE 13.242–244)

This phenomenon of the compulsive unconscious reproduction of an archaic emotional pattern, which Freud called transference and which he saw both as the energetic spring and as the interpretive key to the psychoanalytic situation, is further thought out by Lacan as what accounts for the functioning of authority in general: as essential, thus, not just to any pedagogic situation but to the problematics of knowledge as such. "As soon as there is somewhere a subject presumed to know, there is transference," writes Lacan (S XI.210).

Since "transference is the acting-out of the reality of the unconscious," teaching is not a purely cognitive, informative experience, it is also an emotional, erotic experience. "I deemed it necessary," insists Lacan, "to support the idea of transference, as indistinguishable from love, with the formula of the subject presumed to know. I cannot fail to underline the new resonance with which this notion of knowledge is endowed. The person in whom I presume knowledge to exist thereby acquires my love" (S xx.64). "Transference *is* love . . . I insist: it is love directed toward, addressed to, knowledge" (*Scilicet* 16).

"Of this subject presumed to know, who," asks Lacan, "can believe himself to be entirely invested? That is not the question. The question, first and foremost, for each subject is how to situate *the place from which he himself addresses* the subject presumed to know?" (S xx.211). Insofar as knowledge is itself a structure of address, cognition is always both motivated and obscured by love; theory, both guided and misguided by an implicit transferential structure.

■ Didactic Psychoanalysis: The Interminable Task

In human relationships, sympathies and antipathies usually provoke a similar emotional response in the person they are addressed to. Transference on "the subject presumed to know"—the analyst or the teacher—may provide a countertransference on the latter's part. The analytic or pedagogical situation may thus degenerate into an imaginary mirror game of love and hate, where each of the participants would unconsciously enact past conflicts and emotions, unwarranted by the current situation and disruptive with respect to the real issues, unsettling the topical stakes of analysis or education.

In order to avoid this typical degeneration, Freud conceived the necessity of a preliminary psychoanalytic training of the subjects presumed to know, a practical didactic training through their own analysis which, giving them insight into their own transferential structure, would later help them understand the students' or the patients' transferential mechanisms and, more important, keep under control their own (avoid being entrapped in counter-transference). "The only appropriate preparation for the profession of educator," suggests Freud, "is a thorough psycho-analytic training . . . The analysis of teachers and educators seems to be a more efficacious prophylactic measure than the analysis of children themselves" (SE 22.150).

While this preliminary training (which has come to be known as "didactic psychoanalysis") is only a recommendation on Freud's part as far as teachers are concerned, it is an absolute requirement and precondition for the habilitation and qualification of the psychoanalyst. In his last and therefore in a sense testamentary essay, "Analysis Terminable and Interminable," Freud writes:

> Among the factors which influence the prospects of analytic treatment and add to its difficulties in the same manner as the resistances, must be reckoned not only the nature of the patient's ego but the individuality of the analyst.
>
> It cannot be disputed that analysts . . . have not invariably come up to the standard of psychical normality to which they wish to educate their patients. Opponents of analysis often point to this fact with scorn and use it as an argument to show the uselessness of analytic exertions. We might reject this criticism as making unjustifiable demands. Analysts are people who have learnt to practice a particular art; alongside of this, they may be allowed to be human beings like anyone else. After all, nobody maintains that a physician is incapable of treating internal diseases if his own internal organs are not sound; on the contrary, it may be argued that there are certain advantages in a man who is himself threatened with tuberculosis specializing in the treatment of persons suffering from that disease . . .
>
> It is reasonable [however] . . . to expect of an analyst, as part of his qualifications, a considerable degree of mental normality and correctness. In addition, he must possess some kind of superiority, so that in certain analytic situations he can act as a model for his patient and in others as a teacher. And finally, we must not forget that the analytic relationship is based on a love of truth—that is, on a recognition of reality—and that it precludes any kind of sham or deceit . . .
>
> It almost looks as if analysis were the third of those "impossible" professions . . . Where is the poor wretch to acquire the ideal qualifications which he will need in his profession? The answer is, in an analysis of himself, with which his prep-

aration for his future activity begins. For practical reasons this analysis can only be short and incomplete . . . It has accomplished its purpose if it gives the learner a firm conviction of the existence of the unconscious, if it enables him . . . to perceive in himself things which would otherwise be incredible to him, and if it shows him a first example of the technique . . . in analytic work. This alone would not suffice for his instruction; but we reckon on the stimuli he has received in his own analysis not ceasing when it ends and on the process of remodelling the ego continuing spontaneously in the analysed subject and making use of all subsequent experiences in this newly-acquired sense. This does in fact happen, and in so far as it happens, it makes the analysed subject qualified to be an analyst. (SE 23.247–249)

Nowhere else does Freud describe so keenly *the revolutionary radicality of the very nature of the teaching* to be derived from the originality of the psychoanalytical experience. The analysand is qualified to be an analyst as of the point at which he understands his own analysis to be inherently unfinished, incomplete, as of the point, that is, at which he settles into his own didactic analysis— or his own analytical apprenticeship—as fundamentally interminable.[9] It is, in other words, as of the moment the student recognizes that *learning has no term,* that he can himself become a teacher, assume the position of teacher. But the position of the teacher is itself the position of the one who learns, of the one who teaches nothing other than the way he learns. The subject of teaching is interminably—a student; the subject of teaching is interminably— a learning. This is the most radical, perhaps the most far-reaching insight psychoanalysis can give us into pedagogy.

Freud pushes this original understanding of what pedagogy is to its logical limit. Speaking of the defensive tendency of psychoanalysts "to divert the implications and demands of analysis from themselves (probably by directing them on to other people)"—of the analysts' tendency "to withdraw from the critical and corrective influence of analysis"—as well as of the temptation of power threatening them in the very exercise of their profession, Freud enjoins:

Every analyst should periodically—at intervals of five years or so—submit himself to analysis once more, without feeling ashamed of taking this step. This would mean, then, that not only the therapeutic analysis of patients but his own analysis would change from a terminable into an interminable task. (SE 23.249)

Of all Freud's followers, Lacan has, more than others, picked up on the radicality of Freud's pedagogical concern with didactic psychoanalysis, not only as a subsidiary technical, pragmatic question (how should analysts be trained?) but as a major theoretical concern, as a major pedagogical investigation crucial to the very innovation of psychoanalytic insight. The highly peculiar and surprising style of Lacan's own teaching practice is indeed an answer to Freud's ultimate suggestion—in Lacan's words—"to make psychoanalysis and education (training) collapse into each other" (E 459).

This is the thrust of Lacan's original endeavor both as psychoanalyst and as teacher: "in the field of psychoanalysis," he writes, "what is necessary is the restoration of the identical status of didactic psychoanalysis and of the teaching of psychoanalysis, in their common scientific opening" (E 236). As a result, Lacan considers not just the practical analyses that he—as analyst—directs but his own public teaching, his own Seminar—primarily directed toward the training of analysts—as partaking of didactic psychoanalysis, as itself analytically didactic and didactically analytical, in a new and radical way.

"How can what psychoanalysis teaches us be taught?" Only by continuing, in one's own teaching, one's own interminable didactic analysis. Lacan has willingly transformed himself into the *analysand* of his Seminar so as to teach, precisely, psychoanalysis *as* teaching and teaching *as* psychoanalysis.[10]

Psychoanalysis as teaching and teaching as psychoanalysis radically subvert the demarcation line, the clear-cut opposition, between the analyst and the analysand, between the teacher and the student—showing that what counts in both cases is precisely the transition, the struggle-filled passage from one position to the other. But the passage is itself interminable; it can never be crossed once and for all: "The psychoanalytic act has but to falter slightly, and it is the analyst who becomes the analysand" (*Scilicet* 47). Lacan thus denounces "the reactionary principle" of the professional belief in "the duality of the one who suffers and the one who cures, " in "the opposition between the one who knows and the one who does not know. . . . The most corrupting of comforts is intellectual comfort, just as one's worst corruption is the belief that one is better" (E 403).

Lacan's well-known polemical and controversial stance—his critique of psychoanalysis—itself partakes, then, of his understanding of the pedagogical imperative of didactic psychoanalysis. Lacan's original endeavor is to submit the whole discipline of psychoanalysis to what Freud called "the critical and corrective influence of analysis." Through Lacan we can understand that the psychoanalytic discipline is an unprecedented one in that its teaching does not just reflect upon itself but turns back upon itself so as to subvert itself, and truly teaches only insofar as it subverts itself. Psychoanalytic teaching is pedagogically unique in that it is inherently, interminably, self-critical. Lacan's amazing pedagogical performance thus sets forth the unparalleled example of a teaching whose fecundity is tied up, paradoxically enough, with the inexhaustibility—the interminability—of its self-critical potential.

From didactic analysis, Lacan indeed derives a whole new theoretical (didactic) mode of *self-subversive self-reflection.*

> A question suddenly arises . . . : in the case of the knowledge yielded solely to the subject's mistake, what kind of subject could ever be in a position to know it in advance? (*Scilicet* 38)

> Retain at least what this text, which I have tossed out in your direction, bears witness to: my enterprise does not go beyond the act in which it is caught, and, therefore, its only chance lies in its being mistaken. (*Scilicet* 41)

> This lesson seems to be one that should not have been forgotten, had not psychoanalysis precisely taught us that it is, as such, forgettable. (E 232)

Always submitting analysis itself to the instruction of an unexpected analytic turn of the screw, to the surprise of an additional reflexive turn, of an additional self-subversive ironic twist, didactic analysis becomes for Lacan what might be called a *style.* A teaching style has become at once a life style and a writing style: "the ironic style of calling into question the very foundations of the discipline" (E 238).

Any return to Freud founding a teaching worthy of the name will occur only on that pathway where truth . . . becomes manifest in the revolutions of culture. That pathway is the only training we can claim to transmit to those who follow us. It is called—a style. (E 458)

Didactic analysis is thus invested by Lacan not simply with the practical, pragmatic value but with the theoretical significance— the allegorical instruction—of a paradigm: a paradigm, precisely, of the interminability not simply of teaching (learning) and of analyzing (being analyzed) but of the very act of thinking, theorizing: of teaching, analyzing, thinking, theorizing, in such a way as to make of psychoanalysis "what it has never ceased to be: an act that is yet to come" (*Scilicet* 9).

■ Teaching as a Literary Genre

Among so many other things, Lacan and Freud teach us teaching, teach us what it might mean to teach. Their lesson and their pedagogical performance profoundly renew at once the meaning and the status of the very act of teaching. If they are both such extraordinarily creative teachers, it is—I would suggest—because they both are, above all, quite extraordinarily creative learners. In Freud's case the creative teaching stems from Freud's original (unique) position as a student; in Lacan's case, the creative teaching stems from Lacan's original (unique) position as disciple.

"One might feel tempted," writes Freud, "to agree with the philosophers and the psychiatrists and, like them, rule out the problem of dream-interpretation as a purely fanciful task. But I have been taught better" (SE 4.100). *By whom* has Freud been taught—taught better than by "the judgment of the prevalent science of today," better than by the established scholarly authorities of philosophy and psychiatry? Freud has been taught by dreams: his own and those of others. Freud has been taught by his own patients: "My patients . . . told me their dreams and so taught me" (SE 6.100–101).

Having thus been taught by dreams, as well as by his patients, that—contrary to the established scholarly opinion—dreams do have meaning, Freud is further taught by a literary text:

This discovery is confirmed by a legend that has come down to us from antiquity . . .

While the poet . . . brings to light the guilt of Oedipus, he is at the same time compelling us to recognize our own inner minds . . .

Like Oedipus, we live in ignorance of these wishes . . . and after their revelation, we may all of us well seek to close our eyes to the scenes of our childhood. (SE 6.261–263)

"But I have been taught better." What is unique about Freud's position as a student is that he learns from, or puts in the position of his teacher, the least authoritative sources of information that can be imagined: he knows how to derive a teaching, or a lesson, from the very unreliability—the very *nonauthority*—of literature, of dreams, of patients. For the first time in the history of learning, Freud has scientific recourse to a knowledge that is not authoritative, not that of a master, a knowledge that does not know what it knows and is thus *not in possession of itself.*

Such, precisely, is the essence of literary knowledge. "I went to the poets," says Socrates. "I took them some of the most elaborate passages in their own writings, and asked them what was the meaning of them—thinking that they would teach me something. Will you believe me? I am almost ashamed to confess the truth, but I must say that there is hardly a person present who would not have talked better about their poetry than they did themselves. Then I knew that not by wisdom do poets write poetry, but by a sort of genius or inspiration; they are like diviners or soothsayers who also say many fine things, but do not understand the meaning of them."[11] From a philosophical perspective, knowledge is mastery—that which masters its own meaning. Unlike Hegelian philosophy, which *believes it knows all that there is to know;* unlike Socratic (or contemporary post-Nietzschean) philosophy, which *believes it knows it does not know*—literature, for its part, *knows it knows but does not know the meaning of its knowledge,* does not know *what* it knows. For the first time, then, Freud gives authority to the instruction of a knowledge that does not know its own meaning, to a knowledge (of dreams, of patients, of Greek tragedy) that we might define as literary: knowledge that is not in mastery of itself.

Lacan has best understood and emphasized the radical significance of Freud's indebtedness to literature: the role played by literary knowledge not just in the historical constitution of psychoanalysis, but in the very actuality of the psychoanalytic act, of the psychoanalytic (ongoing) work of learning and teaching. Lacan has best understood and pointed out the ways in which Freud's teaching—in all senses of the word—is not accidentally but radically and fundamentally a literary teaching. Speaking of the training of future analysts, Lacan writes:

> One has only to turn the pages of his works for it to become abundantly clear that Freud regarded a study . . . of the res-onances . . . of literature and of the significations involved in works of art as necessary to an understanding of the text of our experience. Indeed, Freud himself is a striking instance of his own belief: he derived his inspiration, his ways of thinking and his technical weapons, from just such a study. But he also regarded it as a necessary condition in any teaching of psy-choanalysis. (E 435, N 144)

> [This new technique of interpretation] would require for its teaching as well as for its learning a profound assimilation of the resources of a language, and especially of those that are concretely realized in its poetic texts. It is well known that Freud was in this position in relation to German literature, which, by virtue of an incomparable translation, can be said to include Shakespeare's plays. Every one of his works bears witness to this, and to the continual recourse he had to it, no less in his technique than in his discovery. (E 295, N 83)

> The psychoanalytic experience has rediscovered in man the imperative of the Word as the law that has formed him in its image. It manipulates the poetic function of language to give to his desire its symbolic mediation. (E 322, N 106)

> Freud had, eminently, this feel for meaning, which accounts for the fact that any of his works, *The Three Caskets,* for instance, gives the reader the impression that it is written by a soothsayer, that it is guided by that kind of meaning which is of the order of poetic inspiration. (S II.353)

It is in this sense that Lacan can be regarded as Freud's most informed student. Lacan is the Freudian who has sought to learn from Freud how to learn Freud. Lacan is "taught" by Freud in much the same way Freud is "taught" by dreams. Lacan reads Freud in much the same way Freud reads *Oedipus the King*, specifically seeking in the text its *literary knowledge*. From Freud as teacher, suggests Lacan, we should learn to derive that kind of *literary teaching* he himself derived in an unprecedented way from literary texts. Freud's text should thus itself be read as a poetic text:

> the notion of the death instinct involves a basic irony, since its meaning has to be sought in the conjunction of two contrary terms: instinct . . . being the law that governs . . . a cycle of behavior whose goal is the accomplishment of a vital function; and death appearing first of all as the destruction of life . . .
>
> This notion must be approached through its resonances in what I shall call *the poetics of the Freudian corpus,* the first way of access to the penetration of its meaning, and the essential dimension, from the origins of the work to the apogee marked in it by this notion, for an understanding of its dialectical repercussions. (E 316–37, N 101–102)

It is here, in conjunction with Lacan's way of relating to Freud's literary teaching and of learning from Freud's literary knowledge, that we touch upon the historical uniqueness of Lacan's position as disciple, and can thus attempt to understand the way in which this pedagogically unique discipleship accounts for Lacan's originality as a teacher.

"As Plato pointed out long ago," says Lacan, "it is not at all necessary that the poet know what he is doing; in fact, it is preferable that he not know. That is what gives a primordial value to what he does. We can only bow our heads before it" (Seminar, 9 April 1974, unpublished). Although apparently Lacan seems to espouse Plato's position, his real pedagogical stance is, in more than one way, at the antipodes of Plato's; and not just because he bows his head to poets whereas Plato casts them out of the Republic. If Freud himself bears witness to some poetic knowledge, it is to the extent that, like the poets, he too cannot exhaust the meaning of his text—he too partakes of the poetic ignorance of his own knowledge. Unlike Plato who, from his position as an admiring disciple, reports Socrates' assertion of his ignorance without—it might be assumed—really believing in the nonironic truth of that assertion ("For the hearers," says Socrates, "always imagine that I myself possess the wisdom I find wanting in others"), Lacan can be said to be a unique disciple in that he *does indeed, as a disciple, believe in the ignorance of his teacher, of his master.* Paradoxically, this is why he can be said to be Freud's most informed student: a student of Freud's own revolutionary way of learning, of Freud's own unique position as the unprecedented student of unauthorized, unmastered knowledge. "The truth of the subject," says Lacan, "even when he is the position of a master, is not in himself" (S XI.10).

> [Freud's] texts, to which for the past . . . years I have devoted a two-hour seminar every Wednesday . . . without having covered a quarter of the total . . . have given me, and those who have attended my seminars, the surprise of genuine discoveries. These discoveries, which range from concepts that have remained unused to clinical details uncovered by our exploration, demonstrate *how far the field investigated by Freud extended beyond the avenues that he left us to tend,* and how little his observation, which sometimes gives an impression of exhaustiveness, was the slave of what he had to demonstrate. Who . . . has not been moved by this research in action, whether in "The Interpretation of Dreams," "The Wolf Man," or "Beyond the Pleasure Principle"? (E 404, N 117; tm)

Commenting on *The Interpretation of Dreams,* Lacan situates in Freud's text the discoverer's own transferential structure, Freud's own unconscious structure of address:

> What polarizes at that moment Freud's discourse, what organizes the whole of Freud's existence, is the conversation with Fliess . . . It is in this dialogue that Freud's self-analysis is realized . . . This vast speech addressed to Fliess will later become the whole written work of Freud.
>
> The conversation of Freud with Fliess, this fundamental discourse, which at that moment is unconscious, is the essential dynamic element [of *The Interpretation of Dreams*]. Why is it unconscious at that moment? Because its significance goes far beyond what both of them, as individuals, can consciously apprehend or understand of it at the moment. As individuals, they are nothing other, after all, than two little erudites who are in the process of exchanging rather weird ideas.

> The discovery of the unconscious, in the full dimension with which it is revealed at the very moment of its historical emergence, is that the scope, the implications of meaning go far beyond the signs manipulated by the individual. As far as signs are concerned, man is always mobilizing many more of them than he knows. (S II.150)

It is to the extent that Lacan precisely teaches us to read in Freud's text (in its textual excess) the signifiers of Freud's ignorance—his ignorance of his own knowledge—that Lacan can be considered Freud's most attentive reader, as well as a compelling teacher of the Freudian pedagogical imperative: the imperative to learn from and through the insight which does not know its own meaning, from and through the knowledge which is not entirely in mastery—in possession—of itself.

This unprecedented literary lesson, which Lacan derives from Freud's revolutionary way of learning and in the light of which he learns Freud, is transformed, in Lacan's own work, into a deliberately literary style of teaching. While—as a subject of praise or controversy—the originality of Lacan's eminently literary, eminently "poetic" style has become a stylistic cause célèbre often commented upon, what has not been understood is the extent to which this style is *pedagogically* poetic: poetic in such a way as to raise, through every answer that it gives, the literary question of its nonmastery of itself. In pushing its own thought beyond the limit of its self-possession, beyond the limitations of its own capacity for mastery; in passing on understanding that does not fully understand what it understands; in teaching, thus, with blindness— with and through the very blindness of its literary knowledge, of insights not entirely transparent to themselves—Lacan's unprecedented *poetic pedagogy* always implicitly opens up onto the infinitely literary, infinitely teaching question: What is the "navel" of my own theoretical dream of understanding?[12] What is the specificity of my incomprehension? What is the riddle I pose here under the guise of knowledge?

> "But what was it that Zarathustra once said to you? That poets lie too much? But Zarathustra too is a poet. Do you believe that in saying this he spoke the truth? Why do you believe that?"

The disciple answered, "I believe in Zarathustra." But Zarathustra shook his head and smiled.[13]

Any return to Freud founding a teaching worthy of the name will occur only on that pathway where truth . . . becomes manifest in the revolutions of culture. That pathway is the only training we can claim to transmit to those who follow us. It is called—a style.

CHAPTER FIVE

Beyond Oedipus:
The Specimen Story
of Psychoanalysis

I

■ "We are forever telling stories about ourselves," writes Roy Schafer in an essay that suggestively defines the crux of the relation between psychoanalysis and narration, between the daily practice of telling stories and the narrative experience at stake in the practice of psychoanalysis:

> We are forever telling stories about ourselves. In telling these stories to others, we may ... be said to perform straightforward narrative actions. In saying that we also tell them to ourselves, however, we are enclosing one story within another ... On this view, the self is a telling ...
>
> Additionally, we are forever telling stories about others ... we narrate others just as we narrate ourselves ... Consequently, telling "others" about "ourselves" is doubly narrative.
>
> Often the stories we tell about ourselves are life-historical or autobiographical; we locate them in the past. For example, we might say, "Until I was fifteen, I was proud of my father" or "I had a totally miserable childhood." These histories are present tellings. The same may be said of the histories we attribute to others. We change many aspects of these histories of self and others as we change, for better or worse, the implied or stated questions to which they are the answers. Personal development may be characterized as change in the questions it is urgent or essential to answer. As a project in personal

development, personal analysis changes the leading questions that one addresses to the tale of one's life and the lives of important others.[1]

Freud indeed changed our understanding of the leading questions underlying his patients' stories. The constitution of psychoanalysis, however, was motivated not just in the patients' need to tell their stories, nor even merely in Freud's way of changing the essential questions that those narrative complaints addressed, but in Freud's unprecedented transformation of narration into theory. In transforming, thus, not just the *questions* of the story but the very *status* of the narrative, in investing the idiosyncrasies of narrative with the generalizing power of a theoretical validity, Freud had a way of telling stories—of telling stories about others and of telling others stories about himself—that made history.

> My dear Wilhelm,
> My self-analysis is the most important thing I have in hand, and promises to be of the greatest value to me, when it is finished . . . If the analysis goes on as I expect, I shall write it all out systematically and lay the results before you. So far I have found nothing completely new, but all the complication to which I am used . . . Only one idea of general value has occurred to me. I have found love of the mother and jealousy of the father in my own case too, and now believe it to be a general phenomenon of early childhood . . . If that is the case, the gripping power of *Oedipus Rex* . . . becomes intelligible . . . The Greek myth seizes on a compulsion which everyone recognizes because he has felt traces of it in himself. Every member of the audience was once a budding Oedipus in phantasy, and this dream-fulfilment played out in reality causes everyone to recoil in horror, with the full measure of repression which separates his infantile from his present state.[2]

■ What Is a Key Narrative?

"Only one idea of general value has occurred to me. I have found love of the mother and jealousy of the father in my own case too." From the *Letters to Fliess* to *The Interpretation of Dreams*, what Freud is instituting is a new way of writing one's autobiography, by transforming personal narration into a pathbreaking theoretical discovery. In the constitution of the theory, however, the discovery that emerges out of the narration is itself referred back to a story that confirms it: the literary drama of the destiny of Oedipus, which, in becoming thus a reference or key narrative—the specimen story of psychoanalysis—situates the validating moment at which the psychoanalytic storytelling turns and returns upon itself, in the unprecedented Freudian narrative-discursive space in which narration becomes theory.

This discovery is confirmed by a legend which has come down to us from classical antiquity: a legend whose profound and universal power to move can only be understood if the hypothesis I have put forward in regard to the psychology of children has an equally universal validity. What I have in mind is the legend of King Oedipus and Sophocles' drama which bears his name . . .

The action of the play consists in nothing other than the process of revealing, with cunning delays and ever-mounting excitement—a process that can be likened to the work of a psycho-analysis—that Oedipus himself is the murderer of Laius, but further that he is the son of the murdered man and of Jocasta . . .

If *Oedipus Rex* moves a modern audience no less than it did the contemporary Greek one . . . there must be something which makes a voice within us ready to recognize the compelling force of destiny in the Oedipus . . . His destiny moves us because it might have been ours—because the oracle laid the same curse upon us before our birth as upon him. It is the fate of all of us, perhaps, to direct our first sexual impulse towards our mother and our first hatred and our first murderous wish against our father. Our dreams convince us that this is so. King Oedipus, who slew his father Laius and married his mother Jocasta, merely shows us the fulfilment of our childhood wishes . . . While the poet . . . brings to light the guilt of Oedipus, he is at the same time compelling us to recognize our own inner minds, in which those same impulses, though suppressed, are still to be found. (SE 4.261–263)

Freud's reference to the Oedipus as a key narrative is structured by three questions that support his analytical interrogation:

The question of the effectiveness of the story. Why is the story so compelling? How to account for the story's practical effect on the audience—its power to elicit affect, its symbolic efficacy?

The question of the recognition. The story has power over us because it "is compelling us to recognize" something in ourselves. What is it that the story is compelling us to recognize? What is at stake in the recognition?

The question of the validity of the hypothesis or theory. "A legend whose profound and universal power to move can only be understood if the hypothesis I have put forward in regard to the psychology of children has an equally universal validity."

Any further inquiry into the significance of the Oedipus story in psychoanalytic theory and practice, would have to take into account the implications of those three questions: the narrative's practical efficacy (and hence, its potential for a clinical efficacy: its practical effect on us, having to do not necessarily with what the story means but with what it does to us); the meaning of the theoretical recognition (what do we recognize when we recognize the Oedipus?); and the very status of the theoretical validation through a narrative, that is, the question of the relationship between truth and fiction in psychoanalysis.

I would suggest now that Lacan's reading of Freud renews each of these questions in some crucial ways; and that an exploration of this renewal—an exploration of the way in which the Oedipus mythic reference holds the key to a Lacanian psychoanalytic understanding—may hold the key in turn to the crux of Lacan's innovative insight into what Freud discovered and, consequently, into what psychoanalysis is all about.

■ The Complexity of the Complex

Nowhere in Lacan's writings is there any systematic exposition of his specific understanding of the significance of Oedipus. As is often the case, Lacan's insight has to be derived, through a reading labor, from an elliptical and fragmentary text, from sporadic comments, from episodic highlights of (often critical and corrective) interpretations, and from the omnipresent literary usage of the reference to the Oedipus myth in Lacan's own rhetoric and style. My attempt at a creative systematization of what may be called Lacan's revision of the Oedipus mythic reference would organize itself, in a structure of its own, as a relation between three dimensions. (1) *The purely theoretical dimension:* How does Lacan understand the basic psychoanalytic concept of "the Oedipus complex"? (2) *The practical and clinical dimension:* What is, in Lacan's eyes, the practical relevance of Oedipus to the clinical event, to practical dealings with a patient? (3) *The literary dimension:* How does Lacan understand the way in which Sophocles' text informs psychoanalytic knowledge?

Traditionally, the Oedipus complex is understood to mean the literal genesis and the literal objects of man's primordial desire: an incestuous sexual love for the mother and a jealous, murderous impulse toward the father. In this view, what Freud discovered in the Oedipus is a universal *answer* to the question: What does man unconsciously desire? This answer guarantees a knowledge—psychoanalytic knowledge—of the instinctual content of the human unconscious, which can be found everywhere. Any Freudian reading is bound to uncover the same meaning, the ultimate signified of human desire: the Oedipus complex.

This is not the way Lacan understands the gist of Freud's discovery. For Lacan, the Oedipus complex is not a signified but a signifier, not a meaning but a structure. What Freud discovered in the Oedipus myth is not an answer but *the structure of a question,* not any given knowledge but a structuring positioning of the analyst's own ignorance of his patient's unconscious. "If it is true," writes Lacan, "that our knowledge comes to the rescue of the ignorance of the analysand, it is no less true that we too are plunged in ignorance, insofar as we are ignorant of the symbolic constellation underlying the unconscious of the subject. In addition, this constellation always has to be conceived as structured, and structured according to an order which is *complex*" (S 1.78–79). What is essential, in Lacan's eyes, is the key word "complex" in the notion of the Oedipus complex. The fecundity of Freud's paradigmatic schema lies precisely in its irreducible complexity.

When we go toward the discovery of the unconscious, what we encounter are situations which are structured, organized, complex. Of these situations, Freud has given us the first model, the standard, in the Oedipus complex . . . [What we have to realize is] the extent to which the Oedipus complex poses problems, and how many ambiguities it encompasses. The

> whole development of analysis, in fact, was brought about by
> the successive emphases placed upon each of the tensions im-
> plied in this triangular system. This alone forces us to see in
> it an altogether different thing than this massive bloc summed
> up by the classical formula—sexual desire for the mother,
> rivalry with the father. (S 1.79)

The triangular structure, crucial to Lacan's conception, is not the simple psychological triangle of love and rivalry, but a socio-symbolic structural positioning of the child in a complex constellation of alliance (family, elementary social cell) in which the combination of desire and a Law prohibiting desire is regulated, through a linguistic structure of exchange, into a repetitive process of re-placement—of substitution—of symbolic objects (substitutes) of desire.

In this symbolic constellation, the mother's function differs from the father's function. The mother (or the *mother's image*) stands for the first object of the child's narcissistic attachment (an object and an image of the child's self-love, or love for his own body—for his own image), inaugurating a type of mirroring relationship that Lacan calls "the Imaginary." The father (or the *father's name*), as a symbol of the Law of incest prohibition, stands on the other hand for the first authoritative "no," the first social imperative of renunciation, inaugurating, through this castration of the child's original desire, both the necessity of repression and the process of symbolic substitution of objects of desire, which Lacan calls "the Symbolic." While the child is learning how to speak, signifiers of incestuous desire are repressed, become unspeakable, and the desire is displaced onto substitutive signifiers of desire. This is what the Oedipus complex mythically, schematically, accounts for: the con-stitution of the Symbolic, through the coincidence of the child's introduction into language and of the constitution of his (linguistic) unconscious.

The triangularity of the Oedipal structure is thus crucial in La-can's perception in that it implies a radical asymmetry between the Imaginary (archetypal relation to the mother) and the Symbolic (archetypal relation to the structure of alliance between mother, father, and child). The Imaginary is the dual perspective (narcissistic mirroring, exchangeability of self and other); the Symbolic is the triangular perspective. Both are encompassed by the Oedipal structure and will continue to define different registers of human experience and relationships.

> You are familiar with the profoundly asymmetrical character . . . of each of the dual relations which the Oedipal structure encompasses. The relation which links the subject to the mother is distinct from the relation which links him to the father, the narcissistic or imaginary relation to the father is distinct from the symbolic relation, and is also distinct from the relation which we must call real—and which is residual with respect to the architecture which interests us in analysis. All this is enough of a demonstration of the complexity of the structure. (S 1.79)

What matters, in Lacan's perception of the Oedipus as constitutive of the qualitative difference between the Imaginary and the Symbolic, is the fact that the triangularity of the Symbolic narratively functions as the story of the subversion of the duality of the Imaginary. The Oedipus drama mythcially epitomizes the subversion of the mirroring illusion through the introduction of a difference in the position of a Third: Father, Law, Language, the reality of death, all of which Lacan designates as the Other, constitutive of the unconscious (otherness to oneself) in that it is both subversive of, and radically ex-centric to, the narcissistic, specular relation of self to other and of self to self.

II

■ The Clinical Event

In his first Seminar, Lacan reviews a clinical case history reported by Melanie Klein.[3] The reinterpretation he then offers of Klein's narrative sheds light not just on his particular conception of the Oedipus, but on the clinical relevance of this theoretical conception to psychoanaytic practice. First I will sum up the case by quoting from Klein's own report.

> [The case] is that of a four-year-old boy who, as regards the poverty of his vocabulary and of his intellectual attainments, was on the level of a child of about . . . eighteen months . . . This child, Dick, was largely devoid of affects, and

he was indifferent to the presence or absence of mother or nurse. From the very beginning he had only rarely displayed anxiety, and that in an abnormally small degree ... He had almost no interests, did not play, and had no contact with his environment. For the most part he simply strung sounds in a meaningless way ... When he did speak he generally used his meagre vocabulary in an incorrect way. But it was not that he was unable to make himself intelligible: he had no wish to do so ...

[In the first visit] he had let his nurse go without manifesting any emotion, and had followed me into the room with complete indifference ... just as if I were a piece of furniture ... Dick's behaviour had no meaning or purpose, nor was any affect or anxiety associated with it ...

But he was interested in trains and stations and also in door-handles, doors and the opening and shutting of them ...

I took a big train and put it beside a smaller one and called them "Daddy train" and "Dick-train." Thereupon he picked up the train I called "Dick" and made it roll to the window and said "Station." I explained: "The station is mummy; Dick is going into mummy." Meantime he picked up the train again, but soon ran back into the space between the doors. While I was saying that he was going into dark mummy, he said twice in a questioning way: "Nurse?" I answered: "Nurse is soon coming," and this he repeated and used the words later quite correctly, retaining them in his mind ... In the third analytic hour he behaved in the same way, except that besides running into the hall and between the doors, he also ran behind the chest of drawers. There he was seized with anxiety, and for the first time called me to him ... We see that simultaneously with the appearance of anxiety there had emerged a sense of dependence ... and at the same time he began to be interested in the soothing words "Nurse is coming soon" and, contrary to his usual behaviour, had repeated and remembered them ...

It had been possible for me to gain access to Dick's unconscious by getting into contact with such rudiments of phantasy-life and symbol-formation as he displayed. The result was a diminution of his latent anxiety, so that it was possible for a certain amount of anxiety to become manifest. But this implied that the working-over of this anxiety was beginning by way of the establishment of a symbolic relation to things and objects, and at the same time his epistemophili and aggressive impulses were set in action. Every advance was followed by the release of fresh quantities of anxiety and led to his turning away to some extent from the things with which he had already established an affective relation and which had therefore become objects of anxiety. As he turned away from these he turned towards new objects and his aggressive . . . impulses were directed to these new affective relations in their turn . . . He then transferred his interest from them to fresh things . . . As his interests developed he at the same time enlarged his vocabulary, for he now began to take more and more interest not only in the things themselves but in their names . . .

Hand in hand with this development of interests and an increasingly strong transference to myself, the hitherto lacking object-relation has made its appearance . . .

In general I do not interpret the material until it has found expression in various representations. In this case, however, where the capacity to represent it was almost entirely lacking, I found myself obliged to make my interpretations on the basis of my general knowledge . . . Finding access in this way to his unconscious, I succeeded in activating anxiety and other affects. The representations then became fuller and I soon acquired a more solid foundation for the analysis. (pp. 238–246)

What Lacan seeks to understand in Klein's narrative is, specifically, her clinical usage of Oedipus in the originating moment of the therapeutic intervention. This clinical usage, however, strikes him as highly problematic and ambiguous. Lacan is shocked by the reductive crudity of the initial Oedipal interpretation and, as a clinician, disapproves in principle of such "symbolic extrapolations" (S 1.101), of interpretations having the character of a mechanical imposition by the interpreter. And yet this crude originating moment turns out to have been clinically insightful, since it brought about a spectacular therapeutic process. How can that be understood?

She sticks symbolism into him, little Dick, with the utmost brutality, that Melanie Klein! She begins right away by hitting him with the major interpretations. She throws him into a brutal verbalization of the Oedipus myth, almost as revolting to us as to any reader whatever—*You are the little train, you want to fuck your mother.*

This procedure obviously lends itself to theoretical discussions . . . But it is certain that, as a result of this intervention, something happens. This is what it's all about . . .

This text is precious because it is the text of a therapist, of a woman of experience. She senses things, she cannot be blamed if she cannot always articulate what she senses. (S 1.81)

We have to take Melanie Klein's text for what it is, namely, the account of an experience. (S 1.95)

How does one read, how does one listen to, the practical account of an experience? Lacan's reply is: as an analyst, as a practitioner. Indeed, the paradox of the clinical success of a reductive, elementary interpretation, not only triggers Lacan's interest, but actively enhances his attention to a level that is properly, for him, the analytic level. As a clinician, Lacan is always listening, in the discourse that recounts an experience, for its discrepancies, it ambiguities, its paradoxes. The analytic path is always opened up by something that resists, something that disrupts the continuity of conscious meaning and appears to be incomprehensible.

What counts, when one attempts to elaborate an experience, is less what one does understand than what one does not understand . . . Commenting on a text is the same as doing an analysis. How many times have I pointed it out to those I supervise when they say to me—*I thought I understood that what he meant to say was this, or that*—one of the things we should be watching out for most, is not to understand too much, not to understand more than what there is in the discourse of the subject. Interpreting is an altogether different thing than having the fancy of understanding. One is the opposite of the other. I will even say that it is on the basis of a certain refusal of understanding that we open the door onto psychoanalytic understanding. (S 1.87–88)

It is indeed on the basis of Lacan's own *analytical refusal of understanding*—both of the apparently transparent meaning of the Oedipal clinical intervention and of what it is that Klein does understand—that Lacan will shed new light, both on what the Oedipus myth and on what the clinical event are all about.

In much the same way as Freud, dealing with Oedipus, interrogates specifically the practical effect, the narrative efficacy, of the myth, Lacan, withholding understanding of the meaning of Klein's Oedipal intervention, interrogates specifically its narrative-symbolic efficacy: its productive practical and clinical effect. Why is the story of Oedipus—in the clinical experience as in literature— so effective? The question here again is not what does the story *mean,* but what does the story *do?* Not what is the clinician's statement, but what is the clinical significance, the actual principle of functioning, of her performance? Suspending thus what Klein believes she understands, Lacan asks: What is it that Klein does? What does the clinical event—the clinical advent—consist of? What *happens,* in effect, with Dick?

> What then has Melanie Klein in effect done? (S 1.99)

> What is the specific function of the Kleinien interpretation which presents itself with this character of intrusion, of imposition on the subject? (S 1.88)

■ Projection/Introjection: The Clinical Intervention

In her own account of what happens in the therapeutic process, Melanie Klein talks about Dick's development in terms of his projections and his introjections:

> As his analysis progressed it became clear that in thus throwing [objects] out of the room he was indicating an expulsion, both of the damaged object and of his own sadism . . . which was in this manner projected into the external world. Dick had also discovered the wash-basin as symbolizing the mother's body, and he displayed an extraordinary dread of being wetted with water. He anxiously wiped it off his hand and mine, which he had dipped in as well as his own, and immediately afterwards he showed the same anxiety when urinating. Urine and faeces represented to him injurious and dangerous substances.

> It became clear that in Dick's phantasy faeces, urine and

penis stood for objects with which to attack the mother's body, and were therefore felt to be a source of injury to himself as well. These phantasies contributed to his dread of the contents of his mother's body, and especially of his father's penis which he phantasied as being in her womb. We came to see this phantasied penis and a growing feeling of aggression against it in many forms, the desire to eat and destroy it being specially prominent. For example, on one occasion Dick lifted a toy man to his mouth, gnashed his teeth and said "Tea Daddy," by which he meant "Eat Daddy." He then asked for a drink of water. The introjection of his father's penis proved to be associated with the dread both of it, as of a primitive, harm-inflicting super-ego, and of being punished by the mother thus robbed: dread, that is, of the external and the introjected objects. (pp. 243–244)

It should be remembered that, in Klein's conception, the child's mental universe is produced as a relation to a container—his mother's body—and to the imagined contents of this container. During the progress of his instinctual relationship with his mother, the child proceeds through a series of imaginary incorporations. He can, for example, bite or absorb his mother's body: the style of this incorporation implies the destruction of the object incorporated. Within the maternal body, on the other hand, the child expects to encounter a certain number of objects that he projects as dangerous, because he imaginarily invests them with the same capacity for destruction that he experiences in himself. This is why he will need to emphasize their exteriority by expelling them, rejecting them as dangerous entities, bad objects, feces. But still they will appear threatening to him. In order, then, to overcome the threat, the child will reincorporate or introject the dangerous objects, substituting other objects toward which he will deflect his interest. Different objects of the external world, gradually more diversified and more neutralized, will emerge as the equivalents of the first. These imaginary equations between objects will thus produce, in the child's mental functioning, an alternative mechanism of projection and introjection, expulsion and absorption: an imaginary play between contents and container, inside and ouside, inclusions and exclusions.

It would seem that the mechanisms of projection and introjection, based as they are on the play of symmetry (the mirroring, reversibility, and exchangeability) between inside and outside, are themselves basically symmetrical, inverted mirror images of each other. In her account of Dick's alternative projections and introjections, Klein seems to use the terms in this oppositional-symmetric way, which is in fact the way they are routinely understood in psychoanalytic theory.

Lacan, however, points out a radical asymmetry between projection and introjection, and this asymmetry, in his view, holds the key to the very essence of the therapeutic process and is thus crucial to an understanding of what Klein does as a clinician.

> Dick plays with the container and the contents ... He envisions himself as a little train ... The dark space is immediately assimilated to the inside of his mother's body, in which he takes refuge. What does not happen is the free play, the conjunction between the different forms—real and imaginary—of the objects ...
>
> We are here in a mirroring relation. We call it the level of projection. But how should we indicate the correlative of projection? It is necessary to find another term than introjection. In the way we use it in analysis, introjection is not the opposite of projection. It is practically employed, you will notice, only when what is at stake is symbolic introjection. It is always accompanied by a symbolic denomination. *Introjection is always the introjection of the discourse of the Other*, and this fact introduces a dimension altogether different from the dimension of projection. It is around this distinction that you can separate, and see the difference, between the function of the ego, which is of the order of the dual register, and the function of the superego [pertaining to the triangular register]. (S 1.97)

In other words, projection is identified by Lacan with what he calls the (dual) order of the Imaginary. Introjection is understood as pertaining to the (triangular) order of the Symbolic. Projection and introjection are not symmetrical because there is a *qualitative difference* between the Imaginary and the Symbolic. What the therapist does is to introduce this qualitative difference into the child's life, to introduce Dick into the Symbolic (into a symbolic world whereby difference is articulated in a linguistic system), by promoting in the child, all at once, the capacity of *speaking* and the capacity of *substituting* objects of desire, thus permittng him to articulate reality into a symbolic network of differentiated meanings and differentiated object relations.

> You have noticed the lack of contact which Dick experiences ... This is why Melanie Klein distinguishes him from the neurotics, because of his profound indifference, his apathy, his absence. It is clear, in fact, that in Dick what is not symbolized is reality. This young subject is entirely in crude reality, reality unconstituted. He is entirely in the undifferentiated. (S 1.81)

> Anxiety is what is not produced in this subject ... In Melanie Klein's office, there is for Dick neither other nor self; there is reality pure and simple. The interval between two doors is his mother's body. The trains and all the rest are something, without doubt, but something which is neither nameable nor named.
>
> It is against this background that Melanie Klein, with this brute's instinct which characterizes her and which has, incidentally, made her perforate a sum of knowledge hitherto impenetrable, dares speak to him—speak to a being who ... in the symbolic sense of the term, does not answer. He is there as if she did not exist, as if she were a piece of furniture. And nevertheless she speaks to him. She literally gives name to what—until then has been, for this subject, nothing but reality pure and simple—certainly, he already has a certain apprehension of some syllables, but ... he does not assume them. (S 1.82–83)

What drives a child to assume—that is, to endorse, make his, to take upon himself—the vocables of language? In Lacan's conception, the Symbolic—the desire and ability to symbolize—hinges on the more fundamental *need to call:* the need to *address* the other, to attempt to draw the attention of the other toward something that the caller, the addressor, lacks.

> If we sum up everything that Melanie Klein describes of Dick's attitude, the significant point is simply this—the child does not address any call to anybody.
>
> The call takes its value within a system of language which

is already acquired. Now, what is here at stake is that this child emits no call. The system by means of which the subject comes to situate himself in language is interrupted, at the level of speech. Speech and language are not the same; this child is, to a certain extent, master of language, but he does not speak. It is a subject who is there and who, literally, does not answer.

Speech has not come to him. Language has not encroached on his imaginary system . . . For him, the Real and the Imaginary are the same . . .

Melanie Klein does not proceed here—and she is aware of it—to any interpretation. She starts out, as she tells us, with ideas that she has, and which are known . . . Let me make no bones about it, I tell Dick, *Dick–little train, Daddy–big train.* Thereupon, the child begins to play with his little train, and he says the word *station.* This is a crucial moment, in which what is beginning to take place is the encroachment of language on the imaginary of the subject.

Melanie Klein sends him back this—*The station is mummy; Dick is going into mummy.* As of this moment, everything is set in motion. She will give him only statements of this kind, and not others. And very quickly the child progresses. It's a fact.

What then has Melanie Klein in effect done? Nothing other than to provide verbalization. She has symbolized an effective relation, the relation of a being, named, with another. She has applied—indeed mechanically imposed—the symbolization of the Oedipus myth, to call it by its name. It is as a result of that that, after a first ceremony in which the child seeks shelter in the dark space in order to renew contact with the container, something new awakens in him.

The child verbalizes a first call—a spoken call. He asks for his nurse, with whom he had entered and whose departure he had taken as though nothing were the matter. For the first time, he produces a reaction of appeal, of call—a call which is not just an emotional address . . . but a verbalized address, and which henceforth entails an answer.

Things develop consequently to a point where, in a situation henceforth organized, Melanie Klein can bring about the intervention of other situational elements, including that of the father, who comes to play his role. Outside of the sessions, Klein tells us, the relationships of the child develop on the level of the Oedipus. The child symbolizes the reality surrounding him out of this kernel, of this palpitating cell of symbolism which Melanie Klein has provided him with.

This is what she calls, later on, "having opened the doors of his unconscious." (S 1.98–100)

The important point, in Lacan's account of the clinical event, is the following: the initial sentence of the clinician ("Dick–little train, Daddy–big train, Dick is going into mummy") does not function *constatively* (as a truth report, with respect to the reality of the situation) but *performatively* (as a speech act). The success of the interpretation, its clinical efficacy, does not proceed from the accuracy of its meaning ("You want to fuck your mother") but from the way this discourse of the Other situates the child, in language, in relation to the people who surround him, are close to him. This is what the Oedipal intervention is all about. "Melanie Klein does not proceed here to any interpretation," insists Lacan. What the preconceived and heavy-handed interpretation does is to give the child—through the verbalized Oedipal constellation—not a meaning but a *structure,* a linguistic structure by which to relate himself to other human beings; a structure, therefore, in which meaning—sexual meaning—can later be articulated and inscribed.

Let me try to recapitulate the complexity of Lacan's restatement of Klein's clinical account, by stating Lacan's insight in my own terms. After Klein, after Lacan, in the space of insight opened up by the (analytic?) dialogue between their different terminologies, I will sum up in yet another narrative voice the crux of the encounter between Dick and Oedipus.

■ The Story of the Introduction of a Difference

Dick's recovery is the story of his development, his passage, from projection to introjection, from the Imaginary to the Symbolic, from a stage that precedes the primary identification of the "mirror stage,"[4] to a stage in which the secondary identification of the Oedipus is accomplished, through the child's introjection of the "father's name" and the constitution thereby of his superego.[5]

What Klein describes as projection—the *equation,* in her terms, *between "bad objects" and their substitutes*—Lacan designates as the Imaginary. The Symbolic, as opposed to this, would be the *network of equations between these substitutes.* Language is, precisely, a relation between substitutes. Thus, while projection is always in Lacan's conception the displacement of an image from the "inside" to the "outside," that is, a displacement of any one given object with respect to the ego, introjection is not simply the symmetrical displacement of an object from the outside to the inside, but a movement from the outside to the inside of an object's name, that is, the assumption by the ego of a *relation* between a named object and a system of named objects. Introjection, says Lacan, is always a *linguistic* introjection, in that it is always *the introjection of a relation.*

This is why projection is "imaginary," dual ("here" equals "there," "inside" equals "outside"), whereas introjection is "symbolic," triangular (the relation between "inside," "outside," and "myself"). Since naming an element relates it to a *system*—language—and not simply to *me,* who becomes yet another element in the same system, the Symbolic is the differential situating of the subject in a *third position*; it is at once the place *from which* a dual relation is apprehended, the place *through which* it is articulated, and that which makes the subject (as, precisely, this symbolic, third place) into a linguistic signifier in a system, which thereby permits him to relate symbolically to other signifiers, that is, at once to relate to other humans and to articulate his own desire, his own unconscious, unawares.

What, then, is Dick's story in this conception? Initially, Dick has a separate relation (a relation of projection) to each of his imaginary objects. What Klein does is to articulate the relations of the objects among themselves, Dick being one of the objects in the system: Dick learns to assume himself as such, to assume himself as a signifier.

"Dick–little train, Daddy–big train, Dick is going into mummy." In saying this, Klein takes the relation between Dick and the train and articulates it as a relation between two trains. In this way she introduces Dick into the Symbolic through the constellation of the

Oedipal triangle and brings about Dick's secondary (Oedipal) iden-
tificaton. Here is what happens:

I. *Primary Identification* (Imaginary realm of the Mirror Stage)

Projection

here = there	Two elements are seen as equivalent
inside = outside	from the point of view of one of the
container = contents	elements (visual metaphors, specular
my body = my mother's body	fascination).
= my mirror image	
self = other	

II. *Secondary Identification* (Oedipus, introduction into the Symbolic realm)

Introjection

Incorporation of the father's name, constitution of superego

Setting in motion of the mechanism of repression through a chain of displacement of signifiers

Dick is to Mummy what Daddy is to Mummy

"Little train" is to "station" what "big train" is to "station"

"A" is to "B" what "C" is to "B"

Me:mother :: father:mother

A:B :: C:B

The equivalence is not between two objects but between two relations, in
which the substitution of A (Dick) and C (Daddy) is not accomplished by
resemblance (projective identity) but by a parallel position in a structure
(metonymy, desire).

How should we account now for the salutary emergence of
Dick's anxiety? Anxiety is linked to the Symbolic: it is the way in
which the introjection of the symbolic system *as a whole* makes
itself felt in the subject, when any element in it is disturbed or
displaced. There is no relation at first for Dick between the train
and the space between the doors, until Klein establishes—through
discourse—this relation. The rising anxiety in Dick embodies his
nascent intuition that, in a symbolic system, any element or change
has repercussions in the whole. Dick thus develops anxiety, as he
passes fom *indifference* (everything is equally real) to *difference*
(everything is not equally real; there is imaginary; where the
imaginary is, is undecidable).

Dick's Initial Indifference	*The Advent of Difference*
Lack of affect	Difference emerges and is articulated as sexual difference. Everything is not the same. A change in any element changes the givens of a situation. The subject is subject to the givens of his situation, starting with the fact that his sex is one sex and not another.
Lack of anxiety	
Lack of difference	
No change in any element changes anything because everything is the same.	

Anxiety occurs with the assumption of difference (castration), not simply because of the imaginary fear that something (death, or loss of bodily integrity) might happen to the subject, but because of the symbolic recognition that, since everything is not the same and since every disturbance is reverberated in the whole symbolic constellation, the situational givens that affect the subject do make a difference (meaning).

Dick's story is thus Oedipal, in that it is at one and the same time the story of the child's birth into symbolism (language), the story of the human genesis of anxiety (and thus of meaning), and the story of the introduction of articulated difference.

■ The Analytical Speech Act

"It had been possible for me, in Dick's analysis, to gain access to his unconscious," writes Melanie Klein. What, asks Lacan, is the key—the practical, clinical key—to that access? Unlike Klein, who proposes as the key a whole cognitive theory of the child's Oedipal sadism and of the maturation of his instincts, Lacan believes the key is not cognitive but performative.[6] The key is not in the clinician's understanding, or her meaning, but in her actual speech act:

Is it not insofar as Melanie Klein speaks that something happens? (S 1.88)

She sticks symbolism into him, little Dick, with the utmost brutality. . . . But it is certain that, as a result of this intervention, something happens. This is what it's all about. (S 1.81)

What is at stake in this whole observation—what you have to understand—is the virtue of speech, insofar as *the act of speech* functions in coordination with a preestablished, typical, and in advance, significant, symbolic system. (S 1.103)

What does Klein's speech act consist of if it works in the context of a preestablished, typical symbolic meaning? It consists precisely in effectively producing in the child the call that was lacking, the address that then becomes his motivation for the introjection of human discourse (language).

And how does Klein's speech act produce the call in Dick? By calling him ("Dick–little train"), by naming him within the constellation of a symbolic structure, by thus performatively constituting him, through her own discourse, as a subject.

Ask youselves what the call represents in the field of speech. It represents—the possibility of a refusal. (S 1.102)

But if I call the person to whom I am speaking by whatever name I choose to give him, I intimate to him the subjective function that he will take on again in order to reply to me, even if it is to repudiate this function. (E 300, N 86–87

What I seek in speech is the response—the reply—of the other. What constitutes me as subject is my question. In order to be recognized by the other, I utter what was only in function of what will be. In order to find him, I call him by a name that he must assume or refuse in order to reply to me. (E 299, N 86; tm)

In order to find Dick, Klein calls him by a name that he must then acknowledge—assume or refuse in order to reply to her. And Dick indeed replies, first with a call and later with the articulation of his desire. But the call and the desire, the address and the response, the question and the answer, are not statements (meanings), but performances, speech acts. It is thus not on the level of its statements but on the level of its illocutionary forces that the anlaytic dialogue takes place between the therapist and Dick. But this is, in Lacan's conception, the true thrust of any analyic dialogue: fundamentally, the dialogic psychoanalytic disourse is not so much informative as it is performative.

> Whether it sees itself as an instrument of healing, of training, or of exploration in depth, psychoanalysis has but a single medium: the patient's speech. That this is self-evident is no excuse for our neglecting it. Now, speech is what calls for a reply. (E 247, N 40; tm)

> A reaction is not a reply... There is no reply except for *my* desire ... There is no question except for my anticipation ...
> Henceforth, the decisive function of my own reply [as analyst] appears, and this function is not, as has been said, simply to be received by the subject as acceptance or rejection of his discourse, but really to recognize him or to abolish him as subject. Such is the *responsibility* of the analyst, each time he intervenes by means of speech. (E 300, N 86–87; tm; original italics)

■ The Analyst's Responsibility, or the Function of Interpretation

Each time the analyst speaks, interprets in the analytic situation, he gives something asked of him. What he gives, however, is not a superior understanding, but a reply. The reply addresses not so much what the patient says (or means), but his call. Being fundamentally a reply to the subject's question, to the force of his address, the interpretive gift is not constative (cognitive) but performative: the gift is not so much a gift of truth, of understanding or of meaning: it is, essentially, a gift of language. This is how Lacan accounts for the theoretical clarifications Freud gives to the Rat Man, when the patient had to be "guaranteed before pursuing his discourse":

> The extremely approximative character of the explanations with which Freud gratifies him, so approximative as to appear somewhat crude, is sufficiently instructive: at this point it is clearly not so much a question of doctrine, nor even of indoctrination, but rather of a symbolic gift of speech, pregnant with a secret pact. (E 291, N 78–79)

Speech is in effect a gift of language, and language is not immaterial. It is a subtle body, but body it is. (E 301, N 87)

If interpretation is a gift of language—that is, a reply to the analysand's address—rather than a gift of truth, how does interpretation function? If, moreover, in Lacan's conception, "the question of correctness" of the psychoanalytical interpretation "moves into the background" (E 300, N 87), how does the analyst's interpretive intervention bring about the desired therapeutic, clinical effect? Lacan's reply is twofold.

First, since the analyst's interpretation has to be not necessarily correct but *resonant* (ambiguous, symbolically suggestive), since "we learn that analysis consists in playing in all the many staves of the score of speech in the registers of language" (E 291, N 79), "every spoken intervention is received by the subject in terms of his structure" (E 300, N 87). The stake of analysis is precisely to identify the symbolic structure in whose terms the interpretations are received, that is, to identify the structure into which the gift of language is translated, to identify the question in whose terms the reply is sought and heard.

The stake of analysis is nothing other than this—to recognize what function the subject assumes in the order of symbolic relations which cover the whole field of human relations, and of which the initial cell is the Oedipus complex, where the assumption of sex is decided. (S 1.80)

This is, then, the first Oedipal stake of analytical interpretation, whereby the analyst's reply to the analysand is not an answer concerning the initial sexual or incestuous relations of the subject (the Oedipus as answer, as a meaning), but a search for the initial question of the subject (the Oedipus as question, as the constitutive speech act of the patient). Since any spoken intervention or interpretation is "received in terms of the subject's structure," the analytical reply thus seeks the structure of the subject's question. This is what the Oedipus consists in, as an object of the analytical interpretation: it defines the analysand's initial *structure of address:*

In order to know how to reply to the subject in analysis, the procedure is to recognize first of all *the place* where his ego is . . . in other words, to know *through whom and for whom the subject poses his question.* So long as this is not known, there will be the risk of a misunderstanding concerning the desire that is there to be recognized and concerning the object to whom this desire is addressed. (E 303, N 89)

In her first spoken intervention, Melanie Klein, to return to her, has precisely defined this initial structure of address for Dick: "she has symbolized an effective relation, that of a being, named, with another" (S 1.100). Let us not forget, however, that Dick's problem as a child was his failure to address: "If we sum up everything that Melanie Klein describes of Dick's attitude, the significant point is simply this—the child does not address any call to anybody." What Klein in effect does through her first spoken intervention (Oedipal interpretation) is thus not simply to identify the child's initial structure of address, but to create it.

This brings us to the second Oedipal stake of the analyst's spoken intervention and to the second function of interpretation in Lacan's conception.

"Not only is every spoken intervention received by the subject in terms of his structure, but the intervention takes on a structuring function in him, by dint of its symbolic form" (E 301, N 87; tm). Thus not only is the analytic dialogue essentially performative (acting through its illocutionary force) rather than informative (acting through its statements or its meanings); the analytical interpretation in itself is a performative (not cognitive) interpretation in that it has a fundamental structuring, transforming function. If analysis is necessarily always a reference to some "other scene," it is to the extent that it takes place on the performative, other scene of language.

> For in its symbolizing function, the intimation of speech is moving towards nothing less than a transformation of the subject to whom it is addressed by means of the link that it establishes with the one who emits it—or, to put it differently, by means of the introduction of a signifier effect. (E 296, N 83; tm)

This is precisely what Klein has accomplished in the Dick case through her spoken intervention, in spite of the "brutality" of her "symbolic extrapolations." The question then becomes how to account for the spectacular clinical success *in spite of* the symbolical extrapolation, *in spite of* what might be seen as the heavy-handedness of the approach, *in spite of* the mechanical character of the interpretive intervention. Who, or what, is responsible for the therapy's success?

■ The Unconscious Is the Discourse of the Other

Let me quote at some length the suggestive way in which Lacan specifically addresses the question of Klein's clinical success:

> In what way has Melanie Klein done anything whatsoever which manifests a grasp of any process whatsoever which would be, in the subject, his unconscious?
>
> She admits it right away: she has done it—she has acted—*out of habit.* Reread this observation and you will see in it a spectacular demonstration of the formula I am always repeating to you—*the unconscious is the discourse of the Other.*
>
> Here is a case in which it is absolutely manifest. In this subject [Dick], there is no unconscious whatsoever. It is Klein's discourse which brutally grafts upon the initial egotistic inertia of the child the first symbolizations of the Oedipal situation . . .
>
> In this dramatic case, in this subject who has not acceded to human reality because he emits no call, what are the effects of the symbolizations introduced by the therapist? They determine an initial position out of which the subject can put into play the imaginary and the real, and conquer his development . . .
>
> The development takes place only insofar as the subject is integrated into a symbolic system, which he practices and in which he asserts himself through the exercise of an authentic speech. It is not even necessary, you will notice, for this speech to be his own. In the couple instantaneously formed—though in its least affective form—between the therapist and the subject, an authentic speech can be generated. Not any speech will do, of course—this is where we see the virtue of the symbolic situation of the Oedipus.
>
> It is really the key—a very reduced key. I would think—as I have already indicated to you—that there is probably a whole set of keys . . . When we study mythology . . . we see that the Oedipus complex is but a tiny detail in an immense myth. The

myth enables us to collate a series of relations between subjects, in comparison with whose complexity and wealth the Oedipus appears to be such an abridged edition that, in the final analysis, it is not always utilizable.

But no matter. We analysts have so far contented ourselves with it. We are totally mixed up, however, if we do not distinguish between the imaginary, the symbolic, and the real. (S I.100–101)

In this "reduced key" that Freud has named after the story of Oedipus, it is important to distinguish the Symbolic from the Real and from the Imaginary because psychoanalytic practice—that is, psychoanalytic *work*—has to do with the Symbolic. The narrative/symbolic efficacy of the Oedipal reference in the psychoanalytic situation and the therapeutic, practical felicity of the analyst's speech act are accounted for by the resonant and enigmatic formula: "the unconscious is the discourse of the Other." What, precisely, does that mean? And how, specifically, does this formula account for what happens in the Dick case?

In general, when Lacan repeats this formula, what he wants to emphasize, by way of "intimation," are the following key points:

The unconscious is a discourse. Freud is not the first to have discovered the unconscious, but the first to have discovered the essential fact that *the unconscious speaks:* in slips of the tongue, in dreams, in the symbolic language of the symptoms. The unconscious is not simply a forgotten or rejected bag of instincts, but an indestructible infantile desire whose repression means that it has become symbolically unrecognizable, since it is differentially articulated through rhetorical displacements (object substitutions). Repression is, in other words, the rejection not of instincts but of symbols, or of signifiers: their rejection through their replacement, the displacement or the transference of their original libidinal meaning onto other signifiers.

The unconscious is a discourse that is other, or ex-centric, to the discourse of a self. It is in effect a discourse that is other to itself, not in possession of itself; a discourse that no consciousness can master and that no speaking subject can assume or own.

The unconscious is a discourse that is radically intersubjective. Since it is a discourse that no consciousness can own, the only way a consciousness can hear it is as coming from the Other. In this way, the formula describes the analytic situation as coincident with the radical structure of the unconscious, that is, the analytic (dialogic) situation as the condition of possibility for the production of psychoanalytic truth (an audible speech of the unconscious). "The Other" thus stands in the psychoanalytic dialogue both for the position of the analyst, through whom the subject hears his own unconscious discourse, and for the position of the subject's own unconscious, as other to his self (to his self-image and self-consciousness).

> In language, our message comes to us from the Other, in a reverse form. (E 9)

> The unconscious is that discourse of the Other by which the subject receives, in an inverted form, his own forgotten message. (E 439)

In what sense, then, does Lacan say that the Dick case is a spectacular demonstration of his formula of "the unconscious is the discourse of the Other?" Even as applied to this specific case, the Lacanian utterance has many resonances. In a first sense, it is in effect Klein's discourse (her initial Oedipal interpretation) that actively constitutes Dick's unconscious, that is, determines "an initial [symbolic] position out of which the subject can put into play the imaginary and the real, and conquer his development." The constitution of Dick's unconscious (the mental functioning necessitating and enabling the substitution of objects of desire) is coincident, moreover, with Dick's own introduction into language—a language that precedes him and that comes to him from the Other (represented, here, by the therapist); a language that articulates a pre-established sociocultural symbolic system governed by a Law that structures relationships and into which Dick's own relations must be inscribed.

> The development takes place only insofar as the subject is integrated into a symbolic system, which he practices and in which he asserts himself through the exercise of an authentic speech. It is not even necessary, you will notice, for this speech to be his own.

For Dick, then, the unconscious is the discourse of the Other since it is, quite literally, constituted by Klein's discourse.

But, whereas the key to Dick's unconscious is in Klein's performative interpretation, Klein's interpretation is in turn *not her own*.

In what way has Melanie Klein done anything whatsoever which manifests a grasp of any process whatsoever which would be, in the subject, his unconscious?

She admits it right away: she has done it—she has acted—*out of habit*.

Klein has in effect done nothing other than "mechanically apply" (*plaquer*) "the symbolization of the Oedipus myth." If Klein rejoins, thus, Dick's unconscious, it is not because she truly understands its message or directly hears its discourse, but because she is herself inhabited by the discourse of the Other—inhabited by the discourse of the Oedipus myth—of which she is herself nothing but an unconscious medium when, at a loss with respect to any understanding of the child and "out of habit," she quasi-automatically ventures her mechanical interpretation.

Here we are then, up against the wall, up against the wall of language. We are there exactly in our place, that is to say, on the same side as the patient, and it is on this wall—the same for him as for us—that we are going to attempt a reply to the echo of his speech. (E 316, N 101; tm)

For Klein too, then, even as she acts as therapist, the unconscious is the discourse of the Other: the practitioner speaks out of her own unconscious, out of her own inscription into language. And this is always true in Lacan's conception: the psychoanalytical interpreter is not, himself, in possession of the truth of his interpretation, does not possess, in other words, the unconscious discourse he delivers, because the truth of this unconscious discourse is, as such, radically dialogic (it can only come about, discursively, in analytic dialogue; it is neither in, or of, the analyst, nor in, or of, the patient). "In the couple instantaneously formed . . . between the therapist and the subject [Dick], an authentic speech can be generated."

The unconscious is the discourse of the Other, therefore, to the extent that the "authentic speech of the unconscious" is neither Dick's nor Klein's. The Other is in a position of a Third, in the structure of the psychoanalytic dialogue: it is a locus of unconscious language, sometimes created by the felicitous encounter, by the felicitous structural, verbal coincidence between the unconscious discourse of the analyst and the unconscious discourse of the patient. It is a third, not only because it is neither of the two participants in the analytic dialogue but because, with respect to each of these participants, it is also not the imaginary "other" whom each faces. "The unconscious is the disourse of the Other"—of a Third—in that it is ex-centric to, and subversive of, the specular duality (the seductive, narcissistic mirroring) between analyst and analysand.

> This is the field that our experience polarizes in a relation which is only apparently two-way, for any positing of its structure in merely dual terms is as inadequate to it in theory as it is ruinous for its technique. (E 265, N 56)

> It is to this Other beyond the other that the analyst yields his place by means of the neutrality with which he makes himself . . . neither one nor the other of those present; and if the analyst keeps silent, it is precisely in order to let the Other speak. (E 459)

> It is therefore in the position of a third term that the Freudian discovery of the unconscious becomes clear as to its true grounding. This discovery may simply be formulated in the following terms:
> The unconscious is that part of concrete discourse in so far as it is transindividual, that is, not at the disposal of the subject in reestablishing the continuity of his conscious discourse. (E 258, N 49)

Although Lacan elliptically passes over the relation between the paradoxical triangularity of the psychoanalytic dialogue (a triangularity that distinguishes the psychoanalytic dialogue from any other dialogue), and the structural triangularity he insists on in the Oedipus (as constitutive of the Symbolic), it is clear that the *thirdness* of the term that materializes, in the analytic dialogue, the unconscious as "the discourse of the Other" is itself an implicit, subtle reference to the Oedipus. The paradoxical triangularity of the analytic dialogue is Lacan's elliptical sophisticated, and profound way of *referring* the significance of the psychoanalytic situation to the structural significance he has shed new light on in the Oedipus.

This structural significance can be told as *a narrative of the discovery, precisely, of this structure:* a narrative of the discovery of the structure of the psychoanalytic situation. And this, indeed, is Lacan's specific psychoanalytic story.

This Lacanian story, this particular conception of the narrativity of the psychoanalytic dialogue, is, however, very different from the usual one, which attributes the narration in the analytic dialogue respectively, or successively, to the two agents of the dialogue. Such, for instance, is Roy Schafer's story:

> I shall now attempt to portray this psychoanalytic dialogue in terms of two agents, each narrating or telling something to the other in a rule-governed manner. Psychoanalysis is telling and retelling along psychoanalytic lines: this is the theme and form of the present narration. It is, I think, a story worth telling.[7]

But the Lacanian psychoanalytic story is an altogether different story because the narration happens not between two agents but between three terms, and since it takes place (takes effect) only *through* the emergence of this third—this Other; since the subject of the psychoanalytic narration, in all senses of the word (both its speaking subject and what is being spoken of), is neither the analysand nor the analyst, but the discourse of the Other. The psychoanalytic narrative is nothing other, for Lacan, than the story of, precisely, the discovery of the third participant in the structure of the dialogue. And this dramatic, narrative and structural discovery implicitly refers to Oedipus.

As in Freud's case, though in a somewhat different manner, the (elliptical) Lacanian Oedipus emerges, in its peculiar double status as a psychoanalytic key and as a reference story, as an original relation between narrative and theory, between the static, spatial schema of a structure and the dynamic, temporal movement of a story. For Lacan, in much the same way as for Freud, the Oedipus embodies an unprecedented, revolutionary moment of coincidence between narration and theoretizaton.

But if for Freud the Oedipus embodies the insightful moment of discovery at which the psychoanalytic narration—in passing through the analytic practice and in turning back upon itself—becomes theory, it could be said that for Lacan the Oedipus embodies the insightful moment of discovery at which the psychoanalytic theory—in passing through the analytic practice and in turning back upon itself—becomes narration: unfinished analytic dialogue, or an ongoing story of the discourse of the Other.

III

■ The Literary Reference: Oedipus the King

Thus it is that, while Freud reads Sophocles' text in view of a confirmation of his theory, Lacan rereads the Greek text, after Freud, with an eye to its specific pertinence not to theory but to psychoanalytic practice. Freud had already compared the drama of Oedipus to the process of a practical psychoanalysis:

> The action of the play consists in nothing other than the process of revealing, with cunning delays and ever-mounting excitement—a process that can be likened to the work of a psychoanalysis—that Oedipus himself is the murderer of Laius, but further that he is the son of the murdered man and of Jocasta. (SE 4.262)

But while this comparison between the literary work and the work of the analysand leads Freud to the confirmation of his *theory*—a theory of wish, of wish fulfillment, and of primordial Oedipal desires (incestuous and parricidal)—Lacan's different analytic emphasis on the relevance of Oedipus to the clinician's practice is not so much on wish as on the role of speech, of language, in the play.

As we have seen, what Freud discovered in Oedipus—the unconscious nature of desire—implies, in Lacan's view, a structural relation between language and desire: a desire that articulates itself, substitutively, in a symbolic metonymic language, that is no longer recognizable by the subject.

> The relations between human beings are truly established below the level of consciousness. It is desire which accomplishes the primitive structural organization of the human world, desire inasmuch as it is unconscious. (S 11.262)

> It is always at the juncture of speech, at the level of its apparition, its emergence . . . that the manifestation of desire is

produced. Desire emerges at the moment of its incarnation into speech—it is coincident with the emergence of symbolism. (SII.273)

No wonder, then, that *Oedipus the King,* dramatizing as it does the *primal scene* of desire, in effect takes place on the *other scene* of language. Even more than Klein's case history, *Oedipus the King* is in its turn a spectacular demonstation of the Lacanian formula, "the unconscious is the discourse of the Other": for Oedipus' unconscious is quite literally embodied by the discourse of the Oracle.

> Oedipus' unconscious is nothing other than this fundamental discourse whereby, long since, for all time, Oedipus' history is out there—written, and we know it, but Oedipus is ignorant of it, even as he is played out by it since the beginning. This goes way back—remember how the Oracle frightens his parents, and how he is consequently exposed, rejected. Everything takes place in function of the Oracle and of the fact that Oedipus is truly other than what he realizes as his history— he is the son of Laius and Jocasta, and he starts out his life ignorant of this fact. The whole pulsation of the drama of his destiny, from the beginning to the end, hinges on the veiling of this discourse, which is his reality without his knowing it. (S II.245)

> The unconscious is this subject unknown to the self, misapprehended, misrecognized, by the ego. (S II.59)

The Oedipal question is thus at the center of each practical psychoanalysis, not necessarily as a question addressing analysands' desire for parents but as a question addressing analysands' misapprehension, misrecognition (*méconnaissance*) of their own history.

> The subject's question in no way refers to the results of any specific weaning, abandonment, or vital lack of love or affection; it concerns the subject's history inasmuch as the subject misapprehends, *misrecognizes,* it; this is what the subject's actual conduct is expressing in spite of himself, insofar as he obscurely seeks to *recognize* this history. His life is guided by a problematics which is not that of his life experience, but that of his destiny—that is, what is the meaning, the significance, of his history? What does his life story mean?

> An utterance is the matrix of the misrecognized part of the subject, and this is the specific level of the analytic symptom—a level that is decentered with respect to the individual experience, since it is precisely what the historical text must integrate. (S 11.58)

Can we not then view analysis, indeed, as nothing other than this process of historical integration of the spoken, but misrecognized, part of the subject? To achieve this integration, the subject must, like Oedipus, recognize what he misrecognizes, namely, his desire and his history, inasmuch as they are both unconscious (that is, insofar as his life history differs from what he can know or own as his life story).

> What we teach the subject to recognize as his unconscious is his history—that is to say, we help him to complete the present historization of the facts that have already determined a certain number of historical "turning points" in his existence. But if they have played this role, they did so already as facts of history, that is to say, insofar as they have been recognized in a certain sense or censored in a certain order. (E 261, N 52; tm)

As in Freud's case, the reference of the clinical practice of psychoanalysis to the literary drama of the Oedipus hinges on the central question of the *recognition* (as opposed to what the subject had beforehand censored, misapprehended, or repressed). Recognition is indeed, for Freud as for Lacan, the crucial psychoanalytic stake both of the clinical and of the literary work.

The nature of the recognition is, however, somewhat differently conceived, in Freud's discussion of the Oedipus as validating psychoanalytic theory and in Lacan's discussion of the Oedipus as illuminating psychoanalytic practice. In Freud's analysis, Oedipus recognizes his desire (incest, patricide) as unwittingly fulfilled, whereas Sophocles' reader recognizes in himself the same desire, as repressed. The recognition is thus constative, or cognitive. In Lacan's different emphasis, however, the psychoanalytic recognition is radically tied up with language, with the subject's analytic speech act, and as such its value is less cognitive than performative: it is itself essentially a speech act, whose symbolic action *modifies* the subject's history rather than cerebrally observing or recording it at last correctly.

> To bring the subject to recognize and to name his desire, this is the nature of the efficacious action of analysis. But it is not a question of recognizing something that would have already been there—a given—ready to be captured. In naming it, the subject creates, gives rise to something new, makes something new present in the world. (S 11.267)

> Analysis can have for its goal only the advent of an authentic speech and the realization by the subject of his history, in its relation to a future. (E 302, N 88; tm)

The analytical speech act by which the subject recognizes, and performatively names, his desire and his history (insofar as the misapprehension of the one has structured the other) has to be completed, consummated, by an ultimate analytic act of speech that Lacan calls the *assumption* of one's history, that is, the ultimate acceptance and endorsement of one's destiny, the acknowledgment of responsibility for the discourse of the Other in oneself, as well as the forgiving of this discourse.

> It is certainly this assumption of his history by the subject, in so far as it is constituted by the speech addressed to the other, that constitutes the ground for the new method that Freud called Psychoanalysis. (E 257, N 48)

In Lacan's eyes, however, Oedipus the King, while naming his desire and his history, does not truly assume them; at the end of *Oedipus the King* Oedipus accepts his destiny, but does not accept (forgive) himself. This is why Lacan would like to take us, as he puts it (in a formula once again resonant with many meanings), *beyond* Oedipus: first of all beyond *Oedipus the King* and into Sophocles' tragic sequel, *Oedipus at Colonus*.

> If the tragedy of *Oedipus Rex* is an exemplary literary work, psychoanalysts should also know this *beyond* which is realized by the tragedy of *Oedipus at Colonus*. (S 11.245)

■ Beyond Oedipus:
Oedipus at Colonus

It is only in the sequel that the true assumption of his destiny by Oedipus takes place:

> In *Oedipus at Colonus*, Oedipus says the following sentence: *"Is it now that I am nothing that I am made to be a man?"* This is the end of Oedipus' psychoanalysis—Oedipus' psychoanalysis ends only at Colonus . . . This is the essential moment which gives its whole meaning to his history. (S II.250)

What Lacan refers to is scene 2, which I will quote in two different translations:

OEDIPUS
> And did you think the gods would yet deliver me?

ISMENE
> The present oracles give me that hope.

OEDIPUS
> What oracles are they? What prophecy?

ISMENE
> The people of Thebes shall desire you, for their safety,
> After your death, and even while you live.

OEDIPUS
> What good can such as I bring any man?

ISMENE
> *They say it is in you that they must grow to greatness.*

OEDIPUS
> *Am I made man in the hour when I cease to be?*[8]

• • •

OEDIPUS
> You have some hope then that they [the gods] are concerned
> With my deliverance?

ISMENE
> I have, father.
> The latest sentences of the oracle . . .

OEDIPUS
> How are they worded? What do they prophesy?

ISMENE
> *The oracles declare their strength's in you—*

OEDIPUS
When I am finished, I suppose I am strong![9]

"Is it now that I am nothing that I am made to be a man?" What is it, then, that makes for Oedipus' humanity and strength at the very moment when he is "finished," at the moment when, reduced to nothing, he embodies his forthcoming death? What is it that Oedipus, beyond the recognition of his destiny, here assumes and that exemplifies "the end of his analysis"? He *assumes the Other*—in himself, he assumes his own *relation* to the discourse of the Other, "this subject beyond the subject"(S 11.245); he assumes, in other words, his radical decenterment from his own ego, his own self-image (Oedipus the King) and his own consciousness. And it is this radical acceptance and assumption of his own self-expropriation that embodies, for Lacan, the ultimate meaning of Oedipus' analysis, as well as the profound Oedipal significance of analysis as such.

This significance is historically consummated by Oedipus just when he awaits—and indeed assumes—his death. But this is no mere coincidence: the assumption of one's death is inherent to the analytical assumption. "You will have to read *Oedipus at Colonus.* You will see that the last word of man's relation to this discourse which he does not know is—death" (S 11.245). Why death? Here Lacan is at his most hermetic, his most elliptical. I believe, however, that this ellipsis embodies one of his most profound and important psychoanalytic insights, and I will try—at my own risk—to shed some light on it by continuing, now, the analysis of *Oedipus at Colonus* "beyond" what Lacan explicitly articulates, by using some Lacanian highlights borrowed from other texts (other contexts). Let me first make an explanatory detour.

The Oedipus complex, in its traditional conception, encompasses two fantasized ("imaginary") visions of death: the father's death (imaginary murder) and the subject's own death in return (imaginary castration). The Oedipus is resolved through the child's identification with his father, constituting his superego; in Lacan's terms, the resolution takes place (as we have seen in Dick's case) through the introjection of the father's name (embodying the Law of incest prohibition), which becomes constitutive of the child's unconscious. As the first, archetypal linguistic symbol ("name") that represses, and replaces or displaces, the desire for the mother, the father's name (and consequently, in the chain of linguistic or symbolic substitution, any word or symbol used metaphorically or metonymically, that is, all symbols and all words), in effect incorporates the child's assumption of his own death as a condition—and a metaphor—for his *renunciation*. Since symbolization is coincident with the constitution of the unconscious (the displacement of desire), "the last word of man's relation to this discourse that he does not know"—his unconscious—"is death": to symbolize is to incorporate death in language, *in order to survive*.

> So when we wish to attain in the subject what was before the serial articulations of speech, and what is primordial to the birth of symbols, we find it in death, from which his existence takes on all the meaning it has. (E 320, N 105)

> Thus the symbol manifests itself first of all as the murder of the real thing, and this death constitutes in the subject the eternalization of his desire.
>
> The first symbol in which we recognize humanity in its vestigial traces is the grave, and the intermediary of death can be recognized in every relation through which man is born into the life of his history. (E 319, N 104; tm)

What, now, happens in *Oedipus at Colonus* that is new with respect to the recognition story of *Oedipus the King* (besides the subject's death)? Precisely the fact that Oedipus *is born*, through the assumption of his death (of his radical self-expropriation), *into the life of his history. Oedipus at Colonus* is about the transformation of Oedipus' story into history: it does not tell the drama, it is about the *telling* of the drama. It is, in other words, about the historization of Oedipus' destiny through the symbolization—the transmutation into speech—of the Oedipal desire.

OEDIPUS
   My star was unspeakable.
CHORUS
   Speak!
OEDIPUS
   My child, what can I say to them?
CHORUS
   Answer us, stranger; what is your race,
   Who was your father?

OEDIPUS

   God help me, what will become of me, child?

ANTIGONE

   Tell them; there is no other way.   (scene 1, 89)

OEDIPUS

     Or do you dread
   My strength? My actions? I think not, for I
   Suffered those deeds more than I acted them,
   As I might show if it were fitting here
   To tell my father's and my mother's story ...
   For which you fear me, as I know too well.   (scene 2, 91)

CHORUS

   What evil things have slept since long ago
   It is not sweet to awaken;
   And yet I long to be told—

OEDIPUS

   What?

CHORUS

   Of that heartbreak for which there was no help,
   The pain you have had to suffer.

OEDIPUS

   For kindness' sake, do not open
   My old wound, and my shame.

CHORUS

   It is told everywhere, and never dies;
   I only want to hear it truly told.   (scene 2, 102)

OEDIPUS

   There is, then, nothing left for me to tell
   But my desire; and then the tale is ended.   (scene 3, 105)

MESSENGER

   Citizens, the briefest way to tell you
   Would be to say that Oedipus is no more;
   But what has happened cannot be told so simply—
   It was no simple thing.   (scene 8, 147)

Embodying the linguistic drama—the analytical speech act—of
Oedipus' assumption of his radical expropriation, *Oedipus at Co-*

Ionus thus tells not simply the story of the telling of the story of Oedipus, the drama of symbolization and historization of the Oedipal desire, but *beyond* that ("beyond Oedipus"), as the final verses indicate, the story of the transmutation of Oedipus' death (in all senses of the word, literal and metaphoric) into the symbolic language of the myth.

> The fact that Oedipus is the patronymic hero of the Oedipus complex is not a coincidence. It would have been possible to choose another hero, since all the heroes of Greek mythology have some relation to this myth, which they embody in different forms. . . It is not without reason that Freud was guided toward this particular myth.
>
> Oedipus, in his very life, is entirely this myth. He himself is nothing other than the passage of this myth into existence. (S 11.267–268)

> It is natural that everything would fall on Oedipus, since Oedipus embodies the central knot of speech. (S 11.269)

■ Freud at Colonus

At the same time that *Oedipus at Colonus* dramatizes the "eternalization" of the Oedipal desire through its narrative symbolization, that is, Oedipus' birth into his symbolic *life*, into his historical, mythic *survival*, the later play also embodies something of the order of an Oedipal *death instinct:* Oedipus, himself the victim of a curse and of a consequent parental rejection, pronounces in his turn a mortal curse against his sons. Oedipus' destiny is thus marked by a repetition compulsion, illustrating and rejoining, in Lacan's eyes, Freud's tragic intuition in *Beyond the Pleasure Principle*. Like the later Freud, the later Sophocles narrates, as his ultimate human (psychoanalytic) insight, the conjunction between life and death.

> Oedipus at Colonus, whose entire being resides in the speech formulated by his destiny, concretizes the conjunction between death and life. He lives a life which is made of death, that sort of death which is exactly there, beneath life's surface. This is also where we are guided by this text in which Freud is telling us, "Don't believe that life . . . is made of any force . . . of

progress, life . . . is characterized by nothing other than . . . its capacity for death" . . .

Freud's theory may appear . . . to account for everything, including what relates to death, in the framework of a closed libidinal economy, regulated by the pleasure principle and by the return to equilibrium . . .

The meaning of *Beyond the Pleasure Principle* is that this explanation is insufficient . . . What Freud teaches us through the notion of primordial masochism is that the last word of life, when life has been dispossessed of speech, can only be this ultimate curse which finds expression at the end of *Oedipus at Colonus*. Life does not want to heal . . . What is, moreover, the significance of the healing, of the cure, if not the realization, by the subject, of a speech which comes from elsewhere and by which he is traversed? (S II.271–272)

What Lacan attempts here is obviously not a simple reading of the literary Oedipus in terms of Freud's theory but, rather, a rereading of Freud's theory in terms of the literary Oedipus. Lacan's emphasis, as usual, is corrective with respect to a certain psychoanalytic tradition that tends to disregard Freud's speculations in *Beyond the Pleasure Principle* as "overpessimistic" and "unscientific," not truly belonging in his theory. For Lacan, however, *Beyond the Pleasure Principle* is absolutely crucial to any understanding of psychoanalysis, since it embodies the ultimate riddle that Freud's insight has confronted and attempted to convey:

. . . Freud has bequeathed us his testament on the negative therapeutic reaction.

The key to this mystery, it is said, is in the agency of a primordial masochism, that is, in a pure manifestation of that death instinct whose enigma Freud propounded for us at the climax of his experience.

We cannot turn up our noses at this problem, any more than I can postpone an examination of it here.

For I note the same refusal to accept this culminating point of Freud's doctrine by those who conduct their analysis on the basis of a conception of the ego and by those who, like Reich, go so far in the principle of seeking the ineffable organic expression beyond speech that—[they expect from analysis something like an] orgasmic induction. (E 316, N 101; tm)

In reading Freud across *Oedipus at Colonus,* Lacan is doing much more than to suggest an affinity of subjects between Freud's and Sophocles' later works (the constitutive, structural relation between life and death: primordial masochism, death-instinct, repetition compulsion). Lacan is using the relation between *Oedipus at Colonus* and *Oedipus the King* (the undeniable relation, that is, of the later literary work to the specimen narrative of psychoanalysis) in order to make a claim for the importance of *Beyond the Pleasure Principle. Oedipus at Colonus,* says Lacan, is taking us *beyond Oedipus* in much the same way as Freud is taking us *beyond the pleasure principle.* By this multileveled, densely resonant comparison, Lacan is elliptically, strategically suggesting two things:

First, *Beyond the Pleasure Principle* stands to *The Interpretation of Dreams* (the work in which Freud narrates for the first time his discovery of the significance of *Oedipus the King*) in precisely the same relation in which *Oedipus at Colonus* stands to *Oedipus the King.*

Second, the significance of the rejection of Freud's later text by a certain established psychoanalytic tradition (embodying the consciousness of the psychoanalytic movement, that is, its own perception of itself) is itself part of an Oedipal story: the story, once again, of the *misrecognition*—misapprehension and misreading—of a history and of a discourse.

> The unconscious is that part of the concrete discourse . . . which is not at the disposal of the subject in reestablishing the continuity of his conscious discourse. (E 258, N 490)

> The unconscious is that chapter of my history which is marked by a blank . . . it is the censored chapter. (E 259, N 50)

The Oedipal significance of psychoanalysis' misrecognition of its own discourse, of its own history, can only be seen from Colonus. In confining itself, however, to *Oedipus the King* and to Freud's concomitant discovery of wish fulfillment (as theorized in *The Interpretation of Dreams*), the psychoanalytic movement, far from going—as did Freud—beyond Oedipus, is still living only the last scene of *Oedipus the King,* in repeating consciousness' last gesture of denial: the self-blinding. Lacan, on the other hand, strives to make the psychoanalytic movement recognize what it misrecognizes and thus reintegrate the repressed—the censored Freudian text—into psychoanalytic history and theory.

Why is Freud's *Beyond the Pleasure Principle* so important? Why is it not possible to dispense with this final phase of Freud's thought, in much the same way as it is impossible to dispense with *Oedipus at Colonus?* Because, let us not forget, "Oedipus' analysis *ends* only at Colonus . . . This is the essential moment which gives its whole meaning to his history." In what sense can *Beyond the Pleasure Principle* be said to give its whole meaning to psychoanalytic history? In the sense that what is *beyond* the wish for pleasure—the *compulsion to repeat*—radically displaces the conception both of history and of meaning, both of what history means and of how meaning comes to be and is historicized. This radical displacement of the understanding both of meaning and of temporality (or history), far from being episodic, marginal, or dispensable, is essential both to psychoanalytic theory (what has happened in the subject's past) and to psychoanalytic practice (what is happening in the subject's present: the concrete unfolding of unconscious history in the repetition of the transference [E 318, N 102]). Since the compulsion to repeat is, in Lacan's view, the compulsion to repeat a signifier, *Beyond the Pleasure Principle* holds the key not just to history or to transference but, specifically, to the *textual functioning* of signification, that is, to the insistence of the signifier in a signifying chain (that of a text or of a life).

What, then, is psychoanalysis if not precisely a *life usage of the death instinct*—a practical, productive use of the compulsion to repeat, through a replaying of the symbolic meaning of the death that the subject has repeatedly experienced, and through a recognition and assumption of the meaning of this death (separation, loss) as a symbolic means of the subject's coming to terms not with death but, paradoxically, with life? "The game is already played, the dice are already thrown, with this one exception, that we can take them once more in our hand and throw them once again" (S II.256). This is what a practical psychoanalysis is all about. And this is what Freud tells us in his later speculative narrative, which seeks its way beyond the pleasure principle, beyond his earlier discovery of wish fulfillment, beyond his earlier wish-fulfilling way of dreaming Sophocles.

"The Oedipus complex," says Lacan in one of those suggestive,

richly understated statements (pronounced in an unpublished seminar), "the Oedipus complex is—a dream of Freud's." This apparently transparent sentence is in effect a complex restatement of
the way psychoanalysis is staked in the discovery that *The Interpretation of Dreams* narrates: a complex restatement both of Freud's
discovery of the theory of wish fulfillment as the meaning of dreams
and of Freud's *discovery of the narrative* of Oedipus as validating
the discovery of the theory. It was through his self-analysis, out of
his own dream about his father which revealed to Freud his own
Oedipal complexity, that Freud retrieved the founding, psychoanalytic meaning of the literary Oedipus. "The Oedipus complex is
a dream of Freud's."

Now a dream (to a psychoanalyst, at least) is not the opposite
of truth; but neither is it truth that can be taken literally, at face
value. A dream is what demands interpretation. And interpretation
is what goes *beyond* the dream, even if interpretation is itself nothing more than another dream, that is, not a theory, but still another
(free-associated) narrative, another metaphorical account of the
discourse of the Other.

In this respect, it is noteworthy that *Beyond the Pleasure Principle* was at first conceived by Freud as precisely a rethinking of
his theory of dreams. This is borne out by a paper Freud gave at
the International Psychoanalytic Congress at The Hague (1920)
under the title, "Supplements to the Theory of Dreams," where he
announces his forthcoming publication. Here is how the paper's
goal is summed up in the "author's abstract":

> The speaker dealt with three points touching upon the theory
> of dreams. The first two . . . were concerned with the thesis
> that dreams are wish-fulfilments and brought forward some
> necessary modifications of it . . .
>
> The speaker explained that, alongside the familiar wishful
> dreams and the anxiety dreams which could easily be included
> in the theory, there were grounds for recognizing the existence
> of a third category, to which he gave the name of "punishment
> dreams" . . .
>
> Another class of dreams, however, seemed to the speaker
> to present a more serious exception to the rule that dreams
> are wish-fulfilments. These were the so-called "traumatic"
> dreams. They occur in patients suffering from accidents, but

they also occur during psycho-analyses of neurotics and bring
back to them forgotten traumas of childhood. In connection
with the problem of fitting these dreams into the theory of
wish-fulfilment, the speaker referred to a work shortly to be
published under the title, "Beyond the Pleasure Principle." (SE
18.4)

Beyond the Pleasure Principle is thus itself a sort of differential
repetition of *The Interpretation of Dreams,* in much the same way
as *Oedipus at Colonus* is a differential repetition of *Oedipus the
King.*

Indeed, *The Interpretation of Dreams* is also the story of a riddle,
and of its solution. Oedipus solves, first, the riddle of the Sphinx
(by the answer "Man") and then the riddle of who is responsible
for Laios' murder (by the answer "I, Oedipus"). Freud solves the
riddle of the meaning of the dream (by the answer "Wish fulfillment"). Whereas Oedipus goes from the general, theoretical solution (man) to the singular, narrative solution (I), Freud goes from
the narrative solution (self-analysis, I, Oedipus) to the theoretical
solution (man, wish fulfillment).

The later text, however, in both Freud and Sophocles, is not a
simple "supplement" or sequel to the early work, but its problem-
atization. Both later works address *the riddle generated by, precisely, the solution,* the question constituted by the very answer.
Both works embody the enigma of an excess, a subversive residue,
to (from within) the earlier solution: the enigma of the traumatic
dream,[10] in *Beyond the Pleasure Principle,* insofar as this compulsion to repeat manifested as death instinct is not reducible to (goes
beyond) wish fulfillment; the enigma, in *Oedipus at Colonus,* of
Oedipus' assumption of (the gift inherent in) his own death, of (the
blessing incarnated in) his own radical *self-expropriation,* insofar
as this enigma is not reducible to (goes beyond) Oedipus the King's
ultimate *self-recognition,* amounting to the self-denial and the *self-
appropriation* inherent paradoxically in the final gesture of self-
blinding.

In both Freud and Sophocles, then, the final text narrates *the
return of a riddle.* The author of *Beyond the Pleasure Principle*
talks about (to borrow Lacan's terms) "this mystery . . . that death
instinct whose enigma Freud propounded at the climax of his experience." So too Oedipus at Colonus talks about (to borrow Soph-

ocles' terms) "these things (that) are mysteries, not to be explained." And Oedipus, like Freud, is conveying this residual enigma from the position of a teacher: "Indeed, you know already all that I teach" (scene 7, 146).

This final teaching is, however, dramatized in *Oedipus at Colonus* as a *blessing* Oedipus imparts by the mystery in which his death is destined to be wrapped. Now a blessing is not the gift of a solution (in the manner of Oedipus the King) but nonetheless a gift—of speech. At Colonus, Oedipus ends up presenting, then, not a solution but the paradoxical *gift of an engima:* the gift (of speech, the blessing) of the enigma of his own death. In Sophocles' words, when Oedipus announces at Colonus both the gift of his own death and the return of a riddle, we may assume Lacan is hearing Freud's own words beyond his pleasure principle, in that work where Freud in his turn talks about death as a riddle:

OEDIPUS
    I come to give you something, and the gift
    Is my own beaten self; no feast for the eyes;
    Yet in me is a more lasting grace than beauty.
THESEUS
    What grace is this you say you bring to us?
OEDIPUS
    In time you'll learn, but not immediately.
THESEUS
    How long, then, must we wait to be enlightened?
OEDIPUS
    Until I am dead, and you have buried me.
                       (scene 3, 105–106)

A certain psychoanalytical tradition may have come to the conclusion that it no longer has to "wait to be enlightened," since it may believe it has indeed, in burying *Beyond the Pleasure Principle,* buried Freud. But if Freud is like Oedipus, Oedipus is, paradoxically enough, not buried—not yet buried—since the mystery (the riddle) of his mythic disparition is precisely such that Oedipus does die (or disappears), but without leaving a corpse. And it is Lacan who tells us, in the words of Sophocles' messenger, this essential thing, that Freud is not yet buried:

> Citizens, the briefest way to tell you
> Would be to say that Oedipus is no more;
> But what has happened cannot be told so simply—
> It was no simple thing.

While Freud, as dream interpreter, may have indeed said in the very words of Oedipus,

> There is, then, nothing left for me to tell
> but my desire; and then the tale is ended—

and while psychoanalysts may take Freud at his word—believe, in other words, that in the meaning of the wish fulfillment, in the meaning of Freud's story of desire, *the tale is ended*—Lacan is there to tell us that not only is the tale (Freud's, Oedipus') not ended, but that Freud is bequeathing us *Beyond the Pleasure Principle* so as to give us this ultimate discovery: that the tale has, in effect, *no end*.

■ Lacan at Colonus

Thus it is psychoanalysis itself, and not its object, that is now staked in the literary narrative, in the story of the Oedipus. From the perspective of Colonus, Lacan is telling us, retelling us, the very story of psychoanalysis as *what cannot be told so simply:* "it was no simple thing." The story of psychoanalysis is not just the "not simple" story Freud tells, but the very story of Freud's telling and retelling, the narrative, in other words, of Freud himself as narrator. And Freud as narrator is also far from being, says Lacan, a *simple* narrator.

Indeed, this nonsimplicity of the narration—of Freud's narration of his theory—is crucial to an understanding of the theory itself. If *Beyond the Pleasure Principle* is, like Oedipus, not a simple story, it is to the extent that it is, first and foremost, a *strategic* story. What we have to understand, what Lacan is urging us to recognize in Freud's account, is precisely the thrust of Freud's strategy as narrator: not just what the storyteller means to say but (once again) what the storyteller is doing with, and through, his story.

In the final analysis . . . we can talk adequately about the libido only in a mythic manner . . . This is what is at stake in Freud's text . . .

At what point, at what moment, does Freud talk to us about a *beyond* of the pleasure principle? At a point where the psychoanalysts, engaged in the path that Freud has taught them, believe they know. Freud has told them that desire is sexual desire, and they believe him. (S II.265)

The Freudian experience starts out with a notion which is exactly contrary to the theoretical persepective. It starts out by positing a universe of desire . . .

In the classical, theoretical perspective, there is between subject and object a co-fitting, a cognizance [knowledge, that is, possible adaptation, possible equivalence] . . .

It is in an altogether different register of relations that the Freudian experience is inscribed. Desire is a relation of a being to a lack . . . The libido is the name of what animates the fundamental conflict at the heart of human action . . . Insofar as the libido creates the different stages of the object [oral, anal, etc.], no object would ever again be *it* [of no object can desire ever say, "that's it."] . . .

Desire, a function central to the whole of human experience, is desire of nothing nameable. (S II.260–262)

When Freud maintains that sexual desire is at the heart of human desire, all his followers believe him, believe him so strongly that they persuade themselves that it's all so very *simple,* and that all there remains to do with it is science, the science of sexual desire. It would suffice to remove the obstacles, and it should work all by itself. It would suffice to tell the patient—you don't realize it, but the object is there. This is how, at first, the stake of interpretation is understood.

But the fact is, it doesn't work. At this point—the turning point—it is said that the subject resists. Why? Because Freud has said so. But one has not understood what it means to *resist* any more than one has understood the meaning of *sexual desire.* One believes one has to push. At this point, the analyst himself succumbs to a delusion. I have shown you what the *insistence* means on the part of the suffering subject. Now, the analyst is putting himself at the same level, he too *insists* in his own way, a way which is, however, much more stupid, because conscious . . .

Resistance is . . . the current state of interpretation of the subject. It is the manner in which, at this moment, the subject interprets the point he is at. This resistance is an abstract, ideal point. It is you who call that resistance. It only means that the subject cannot advance more quickly . . .

There is only one resistance, the resistance of the analyst. The analyst resists when he does not understand what is happening in the treatment. He does not understand what is happening in the treatment when he believes that interpreting is showing to the subject that what he desires is such-and-such sexual object. He is mistaken . . . It is he who is in a state of inertia and of resistance.

The psychoanalytic goal is, on the contrary, to teach the subject to name, to articulate, to pass into existence this desire which is, literally, beneath existence, and for that very reason, insists . . .

To bring the subject to recognize and to name his desire, this is the nature of the efficacious action of analysis. But it is not a question of recognizing something that would have already been there—a given . . .

Since, in a sort of balancing, we always place ourselves between the text of Freud and our practical experience, I urge you to return now to Freud's text, so as to realize that the *Beyond* [of the pleasure principle] situates desire, in effect, beyond any instinctual cycle, specifically definable by its conditions. (S 11.266–267)

"In the final analysis, we can talk adequately about the libido only in a mythic manner: this is what is at stake in Freud's text." In *Beyond the Pleasure Principle* Freud creates a new myth—that of the death instinct—so as to demystify the literal belief in, and the simplified interpretation of, his first myth of the Oedipus. Freud is thus essentially a demystifying narrator. But the narrative strategy of *demystification* takes place only through a new narrative *mythification*. In urging us to go *beyond* the myth, Freud also tells us that beyond the myth there is, forever, another myth. And it is in this sense also that the tale (Freud's, Oedipus', Lacan's) is never ended.

But who is speaking here? *Whose irony* is it that traverses the narration of the psychoanalytic story and *unends* the (Oedipal, or Freudian, or Lacanian) tale? Lacan's voice fuses here with Freud's in what Lacan would doubtless call, a "[narrative] inmixture of the subjects"[11]: the story of Freud's strategy as psychoanalytic narrator is simultaneously the story of Lacan as psychoanalytic educator. So that if we ask, "Whose story is it (Freud's? Lacan's? Oedipus'?)?" the answer is not clear. And if we ask, "Whose narrative voice is carrying through this narrative performance (Freud's? Lacan's? Sophocles'?)?" the answer is not clear. But if we ask, "What is this narrative performance doing?" the answer is quite clear. If we ask, that is, in a Lacanian manner, the question not of who is the true *owner* of the story (to whom does it belong?), not of whom Lacan is *quoting* in the story, not of what Lacan *means* by the story, but what Lacan *is doing* with this story, the answer would be unambiguous: Lacan is training analysts. Lacan as narrator of Freud as narrator, Lacan as narrator of Sophocles as narrator, Lacan in everyting he says or does, and in the very way he breathes (breathes texts and breathes psychoanalytic practice), is always, above all, a *training analyst.*

This is why, no doubt, he picks Colonus as the truly psychoanalytic place: for if Colonus—and Colonus only—marks "the end of Oedipus' psychoanalysis," it is to the extent that Oedipus' tale of desire ends only through its own dramatic, narrative discovery that the tale has, in effect, no end: the end of Oedipus' analysis, in other words, is the discovery that analysis, and in particular didactic self-analysis, is interminable. In dramatizing Oedipus' assumption of his own death, of his own expropriating discourse of the Other, and his analytic passage *beyond* his ego, Colonus, as "the end of Oedipus' psychoanalysis," marks the moment at which the analysand beomes an analyst, ready to bestow, indeed, precisely that by which Lacan has characterized the analyst's spoken intervention: a gift of speech. Colonus thus echoes Lacan's preoccupations as a training analyst.

Yet if Colonus resonates so forcefully in Lacan; strikes such a forceful chord in Lacan's insight, it is because Lacan, perhaps unconsciously, identifies with Oedipus at Colonus. While Freud identifies quite naturally with Oedipus the King or the conquistador, the *riddle solver* (who is, incidentally, a father-killer and a mother-lover, king to his own mother), even as he knows that this stupendous riddle solving will bring about "the Plague,"[12] Lacan identifies quite naturally with Oedipus the exile (a survivor of the Plague). We should recall here that Lacan himself, as a training analyst, was expropriated, excommunicated from the International Psychoanalytical Association.

> I am here, in the posture which is mine, in order to always address the same question—What *does psychoanalysis mean?* . . .
>
> The place from which I am readdressing this problem is in effect a place which has changed, which is no longer altogether inside, and of which one does not know whether it is outside.
>
> This reminder is not anecdotal . . . I hand you this, which is a fact—that my teaching, designated as such, has been the object of a quite extraordinary censorship declared by an organism which is called the Executive Committee of an international organization which is called the International Psychoanalytical Association. What is at stake is nothing less than the prohibition of my teaching, which must be considered as null and void insofar as it concerns the habilitation of psychoanalysts; and this proscription has been made the condition for the affiliation of the psychoanalytic society of which I am a member with the International Psychoanalytic Association . . .
>
> What is at stake is, therefore, something of the order of what is called . . . a major excommunication . . .
>
> I believe . . . that not only by the echoes it evokes, but by the very structure it implies, this fact introduces something which is at the very principle of our interrogation concerning psychoanalytic practice. (S XI.9)

Colonus thus embodies, among other things, not just Lacan's own exile, Lacan's own story of expropriation from the Association, but Lacan's dramatic, tragic understanding that psychoanalysis is radically *about expropriation* and his assumption of his story, his assumption, that is, all at once of his own death and of his own myth—of the legacy of this expropriation—as his truly destined psychoanalytic legacy and as his truly training psychoanalytic question: "Is it now that I am nothing that I am made to be a man?"

"It was ordained: I recognize it now," says Oedipus at Colonus. Perhaps we can even hear Lacan's own voice in the very words of Oedipus the exile:

OEDIPUS
That stranger is I. As they say of the blind,
Sounds are the things I see.   (scene 1, 85)

ISMENE
The oracles declare their strength's in you—
OEDIPUS
When I am finished, I suppose I am strong!   (scene 2, 96)

OEDIPUS
I come to give you something, and the gift
Is my own beaten self: no feast for the eyes;
Yet in me is a more lasting grace than beauty.
THESEUS
What grace is this you say you bring to us?
OEDIPUS
In time you'll learn, but not immediately.
THESEUS
How long, then, must we wait to be enlightened?
OEDIPUS
Until I am dead, and you have buried me.   (scene 3, 106)

■ Psychoanalysis at Colonus

As Lacan is talking about Oedipus at Colonus, then, he is telling and retelling not just Freud's, and his own, psychoanalytic story but the very story of psychoanalysis, seen from Colonus: the story of Freud's going beyond Freud, of Oedipus' going beyond Oedipus, the story of psychoanalysis' inherent, radical, and destined self-expropriation. Lacan thus recapitulates at once the meaning of the story in which Freud is taking us beyond his own solution to the riddle, and the narrative voice—or the narrative movement—by which Freud expropriates, in fact, not just his own solution but his own narrative.

In subscribing to Freud's psychoanalytic self-recognition in the

Oedipus, as the moment of psychoanalysis' self-appropriation, its coming into the possession of its "scientific" knowledge, and in censoring *Beyond the Pleasure Principle* as "nonscientific," a certain established psychoanalytical tradition has tried to censor this final Freudian self-expropriation, and this narrative annunciation, by the "father of the psychoanalytic movement," of an inherent *exile of psychoanalysis:* an exile from a nonmythical access to truth; an exile, that is, from any final rest in a knowledge guaranteed by the self-possessed kingdom of a theory, and the constrained departure from this kingdom into an uncertain psychoanalytic *destiny of erring.*

Against this rejection of Freud's text, this repression of the very revolution involved in Freud's narration (in the unprecedented, self-trespassing, self-expropriating status of his narrative), Lacan has raised his training and psychoanalytic voice; but his protestation is then censored in its turn. Whatever the polemical pretexts or the political reasons given by the censors, it is clear that the profound (and perhaps unconscious) thrust of the repressive gesture is the same: to eradicate from psychoanalysis the threat of its own self-expropriation (to repeat the Oedipal gesture of self-blinding); to censor thereby, in Freud as well as in Lacan, the radically self-critical and self-transgressive movement of the psychoanalytic discourse; to pretend, or truly to believe, that this self-transgression and this self-expropriation, far from being the essential, revolutionary feature of the psychoanalytic discourse, is nothing other than a historical accident, one particular historical chapter, easily erased.

However, the repeated psychoanalytic censorships illustrate only the working truth of Freud's *Beyond the Pleasure Principle* (or of Sophocles'/Lacan's *Oedipus at Colonus).* In dramatizing the compulsion to repeat in the very midst of the psychoanalytic institution, they bear witness to the Freudian story, illustrate the Freudian myth of (something like) a death instinct of psychoanalysis itself: the repetition of a curse in a discourse destined to bestow speech as a blessing.

Through his call for "a return to Freud"—*a return to Colonus*—Lacan himself embodies, in the history of the psychoanalytic movement, a return of the repressed. This is why, like Oedipus at Colonus, he too announces (and his entire style is a symptom of this announcement) the return of a riddle.

THESEUS
What grace is this you say you bring to us?
OEDIPUS
In time you'll learn, but not immediately.
THESEUS
How long, then, must we wait to be enlightened?
OEDIPUS
Until I am dead, and you have buried me.

But Lacan's narrative is at the same time a dramatic repetition of the radical impossibility of ever burying the speech of the unconscious. The riddle persists. And so does Lacan's story, whose subject, in all senses of the word, is precisely *the insistence of the riddle.*

What, however, is a riddle if not a narrative delay ("In time you'll learn"), the narrative analytical *negotiation* of some truth or insight, and its metaphorical approximation through a myth? The rejection of *Beyond the Pleasure Principle* under the pretext that, as myth, it is unscientific ("just a myth") involves a misunderstanding both of what a myth is all about and of the status of the myth as such in Freud's narration and in psychoanalytic theory (But, then again, the misrecognition of a myth is what psychoanalysis is all about.) "In the final analysis . . . we can talk adequately about the libido only in a mythic manner . . . This is what is at stake in Freud's text" (S II.265).

In trying to decipher the significance of Freud's work, Lacan insists not only on the significance of Freud's myths but, even more important, on the often overlooked significance of Freud's acknowledgment of his own myths:

At this point I must note that in order to handle any Freudian concept, reading Freud cannot be considered superfluous, even for those concepts that are homonyms of current notions. This has been well demonstrated, I am opportunely reminded, by the misadventure that befell Freud's theory of the instincts, in a revision of Freud's position by an author less than alert to Freud's explicit statement of the mythical status of this theory. (E 246, N 39; tm)

Freud's own terms of acknowledgment of his own myth are indeed enlightening:

The theory of the instincts is so to say our mythology. Instincts are mythical entities, magnificent in their indefiniteness. In our work, we cannot for a moment disregard them, yet we are never sure that we are seeing them clearly. (SE 22.95)

Myth in Freud is not an accident of theory: it is not external to the theory, but the very vehicle of theory, a vehicle of *mediation between practice and theorization.* Freud's complex acknowledgment of the mythic status of his discourse is reflected, echoed, meditated in Lacan's response:

I would like to give you a more precise idea of the manner in which I plan to conduct this seminar.

You have seen, in my last lectures, the beginning of *a reading of what one might call the psychoanalytic myth.* This reading goes in the direction, not so much of criticizing this myth, as of *measuring the scope of the reality* with which it comes to grips, and to which it gives its *mythical reply.* (S 1.24)

The analytical experience, says Lacan, has been involved, since its origins, not simply with fiction but with the "truthful" structural necessity of fiction, that is, with its symbolical nonarbitrariness (E 12,17). Like the analytical experience, the psychoanalytic myth is constituted by "that very truthful fictitious structure" (E 449). Insofar as it is mediated by a myth, the Freudian theory is not a literal translation or reflection of reality, but its *symptom,* its metaphorical account. The myth is not pure fantasy, however, but has narrative symbolic logic that accounts for a real mode of functioning, a real structure of relations. The myth is not reality, but neither is it what it is commonly understood to be—a simple opposite of reality. Between reality and the psychoanalytic myth, the relation is not one of opposition, but one of analytic dialogue: the myth comes to grips with something in reality that it does not fully comprehend but to which it gives an answer, a *symbolic reply.* The function of the myth in psychoanalytic theory is thus evocative of the function of interpretation in the psychoanalytic dialogue: the Freudian mythical account can be thought of as Freud's theoretical gift of speech.

What does that mean? In much the same way as the gift of speech of analytical interpretation, within the situation of the dialogue, acts not by virtue of its accuracy but by virtue of its resonance (received in terms of the listener's structure), works, that is, by virtue of its openness to a linguistic passage through the Other, so does the psychoanalytic myth, *in resonating in the Other,* produce a *truthful structure.* The psychoanalytic myth derives its theoretical effectiveness not from its truth value, but from its truth encounter with the other, from its capacity for *passing through the other;* from its openness, that is, to an *expropriating passage* of one insight through another, of one story through another—the passage, for example, of *Oedipus the King* through *Oedipus at Colonus,* or the passage of the myth of "instinct" through this later and more troubling myth of "death":

> As a moment's reflection shows, the notion of the death instinct involves a basic irony, since its meaning has to be sought in the conjunction of two contrary terms: instinct in its most comprehensive acceptation being the law that governs in its succession a cycle of behaviour whose goal is the accomplishment of a vital function; and death appearing first of all as the destruction of life . . .
>
> This notion must be approached through its *resonances* in what I shall call *the poetics of the Freudian corpus, the first way of access to the penetration of its meaning,* and the essential dimension, from the origins of the work to the apogee marked in it by this notion, for an understanding of its dialectical repercussions. (E 316–317, N 101–102)

> The psychoanalytic experience has discovered in man the imperative of the Word as the law that has formed him in its image. It manipulates the poetic function of language to give to his desire its symbolic mediation. May that experience enable you to understand at last that *it is in the gift of speech that all the reality of its effects resides;* for it is by way of this gift that all reality has come to man and it is by his continued act that he maintains it.

> If the domain defined by this gift of speech is to be sufficient for your action as also for your knowledge, it will also be sufficient for your devotion. (E 322, N 106)

Lacan's involvement with the Freudian myth (viewed as the literary gift of speech accomplished by Freud's discourse, through the dimension of narration in psychoanalytic theory) is thus radically involved with the difference Freud is introducing into the conception and practice of narration, a psychoanalytic difference that Lacan himself is replicating, in his own way, in his own theoretical and mythical gift of speech. Lacan's involvement with the psychoanalytic difference in narration has three aspects: (1) Lacan's narration (both the story that he tells and his narrative voice, or style) is very different from the usual psychoanalytic narration of Freud's accomplishment and theory. (2) Lacan's narration is *about* difference. (3) The psychoanalytic narration, in Lacan's conception (modeled as it is on analytic dialogue), is always different from itself. In the very way it is narrated, the psychoanalytic theory inscribes a radical self-difference. And this self-difference, this *Spaltung* in the theory, this unavoidable breach of theory, *is* the myth. The myth is thus at once the Other of the theory and that which *gives* the theory to itself, that which founds the theory from within the literary gift of speech. While there is no possible cognition of the myth—no constative exhaustion of the myth by theory—there should be a *performative* acknowledgment ("recognition" and "assumption") by the theory of its relation to the myth, and of the irreducibility of the myth, as something in the theory that, paradoxically enough, both expropriates it from its truth and at the same time founds it as "a fictitious truthful structure." The myth is structurally truthful, and psychoanalytically effective, not just in function of but in proportion to its capacity for narrative expropriation.

This is why Freud has privileged the Oedipus above all other myths. In dramatizing language as the acting-out of the unconscious (in both its clinical and its literary implications), the Oedipus is archetypal of the psychoanalytic myth in that it is the story of the narrative expropriation of the story by itself, the story of, precisely, the acknowledgment of the misrecognition of the story by itself. Misleadingly, the Oedipus appears at first to be a myth of possession (of a kingdom, of a woman, of the solution to a riddle, of one's own story). But, as it turns out, the Oedipus is not the myth of the possession of a story, but the myth, precisely, of the dispossession by the story—the dispossession of the possessor of the story. Any kingdom or possession coming out of the psychoanalytic riddle solving is, in fact, incestuous and, as such, is bound to bring about a plague. Psychoanalysis can only be a gift of speech from the exile of Colonus.

As a narrative of this discovery, as a narrative, that is, not just of a discovery but of the discovery of difference, the story of Oedipus exemplifies the psychoanalytic myth in that it exemplifies the problematic status of psychoanalysis telling its own story of discovery and, while telling, acting out its own unconscious. It does something through the telling that the telling fails to account for, and thus discovers and rediscovers the difference between what it is telling and what it is doing in the telling, as the scene of its own dismantling by the literary myth and of its own theoretical self-subversion. The Oedipus is privileged, thus, as a myth not only because it is about the creation of the myth ("Oedipus himself is nothing other than the passage of this myth into existence"), but because it is specifically about the *subversively performative aspect* of this mythical creation. The story of the Oedipus is archetypal of the psychoanalytic myth in that it dramatizes speech not as cognitive but as performative: it embodies this performative self-difference within its own narration, this practical discrepancy, forever reemerging, between its narrative or mythic statement and its narrative or mythical performance.

How, indeed, could speech exhaust the meaning of speech . . . except in the act that engenders it? Thus Goethe's reversal of its presence at the origin of things, "In the beginning was the act," finds itself reversed in its turn: it was certainly the *speech act* that was in the beginning, and we live in its creation, but it is the action of our mind that continues this creation by constantly renewing it. And *we can only turn back on that action by allowing ourselves to continue to be driven by it even further.*

I know only too well that this will be my own case, too, in trying now to turn back upon the act of speech. (E 271, N 61; tm)

■ Beyond Colonus: Truth and Science, or What Remains To Be Narrated

If Freud's psychoanalysis is, then, a symbolic reply to a reality it tries to come to grips with—and if this symbolic reply is made of myth—it is to the extent that, in its function as a gift of speech, the psychoanalytic myth embodies *a residue of action in the very process of cognition* of that action. In another sense, this is also what Freud has talked about: "Instincts are mythical entities, magnificent in their indefiniteness. *In our work we cannot for a moment disregard them; yet we are never sure that we are seeing them clearly."* Myth is something we cannot be sure we are seeing clearly, but we work with it because it works. Myth is thus a mediation between action and cognition, between theory and practice, a narrative negotiation of difference and self-difference in the very practice of a discourse that purports to be cognitive and theoretical. As we have seen in the Oedipus, myth is first and foremost *efficacious, both clinically and literarily.* And it is perhaps because it combines the performative power of the clinical event and the performative power of the literary resonance that the Oedipus has worked so well as the specimen story of psychoanalysis: a specimen story, however, that in the very act of grounding psychoanalytic theory also points to the irreducible expropriating residue of action in cognition, of fiction (narrative) in truth, of practice (dialogue) in theory.

Action, fiction, and practice are thus bound together in the irreducibility of myth from the science of psychoanalysis. For the acknowledgment of the irreducibility of the mythic element in psychoanalytic theory is by no means an abdication, in Lacan's case or in Freud's, of the commitment to psychoanalysis as science. "It may perhaps seem to you," writes Freud, "as though our theories are a kind of mythology and, in the present case, not even an agreeable one": "But does not every science come in the end to a kind of mythology like this? Cannot the same be said of today's physics?" (SE 22.211).

In following Freud's mythical *and* scientific path, Lacan's interrogation, as opposed to Freud's, concerns here again not the theory but the practice. Can the practice of psychoanalysis have a scientific claim? Does the practice work (and if so, how?), out of reference to a truth that is of the order of a science? Lacan replies in the affirmative. But his answer is, as usual, paradoxical and challenging in the way it (analytically) displaces our expectation as to what a science is and where the science of psychoanalysis would reside. If science is involved in the practice of psychoanalysis, it is not because the analyst is scientific, says Lacan, but because the patient is, or can be. Yet the patient is not, as we might expect, the object of the science of psychoanalysis, but its subject. The scientific question of psychoanalysis thus becomes the question of "the subject of science" (E 859), a subject that can be defined by the structure of his (her) "relation to truth as cause" (E 873). This psychoanalytic truth as cause (a cause at once material, formal, and efficacious) is "the incidence of the signifier" (insofar as it has *caused* the subject's unconscious). And this scientific cause is what the subject—the analysand—is after.

> I would like to ask you, analysts, the question: yes or no, does the exercise of your profession have the meaning of affirming that the truth of neurotic suffering is—*to have truth as its cause* [to have a rational causality that, though symbolic, has both a reference to and a bearing on the Real]? (E 870)

> This is why it was important to promote before all else, and as a fact to be distinguished from the question of whether or not psychoanalysis is a science (whether or not its field is scientific)—this fact, precisely, that its praxis implicates no other subject than the subject of science. (E 863)

Contrary to received opinion, Lacan's preoccupation is not with theory per se (with games of "intellectualization"), but always with his practice as a psychoanalytical clinician. He is first and foremost a practitioner, who happens to be thinking about what he is doing in his practice. His *theory* is nothing other than his training practice— his practice as an educator, a training analyst who introduces others to the pragmatic questions of the practice.

Now this commitment to the practice of psychoanalysis as science, together with the acknowledgment that psychoanalytic theory is fundamentally and radically composed of myth—that the knowledge which is theorized out of the practice cannot transgress its status as a *narrative expropriating its secured possession as a knowledge*—has repercussions both in theory and in practice. It means that, to be truly scientific, the practice has to be conceived as antecedent to the knowledge: it has to be forgetful of the knowledge.

> Science, if you look into it, has no memory. It forgets the peripeties out of which it has been born; it has, in other words, a dimension of truth that psychoanalysis puts into practice. (E 869)

[To be a good psychoanalyst is to find oneself] in the heart of a concrete history where a dialogue is engaged, in a register where no sort of truth is reparable in the form of a knowledge which is generalizable and always true. To give the right reply to an event insofar as it is significant is . . . to give a good interpretation. And to give a good interpretation at the right time is to be a good analyst. (S II.31)

Any operation in the field of analytic action is anterior to the constitution of knowledge, which does not preclude the fact that in operating in this field, we have constituted knowledge . . .

For this reason, the more we know, the greater the risks we run. Everything that you are taught in a form more or less predigested in the so-called institutes of psychoanalysis (sadistic, anal stages, etc.) is of course very useful, especially for nonanalysts. It would be stupid for psychoanalysts to systematically neglect it, but they should know that this is not the dimension in which they operate. (S II.30)

The peculiar scientific status of psychoanalytic practice, then, is such that psychoanalysis (as an individual advent and process) is always living and reliving the very moment of the birth of knowledge: the moment, that is, of *the birth of science.* Like Oedipus at the beginning of his mythical itinerary, psychoanalysis has no use for the Oedipus myth insofar as it has entered, through the oracles, the domain of public discourse. Like Oedipus, psychoanalysis has no use for a preconceived knowledge of the mythic story, no use for the story insofar as the story is, precisely, well known in advance. *In practice,* there is no such thing as a specimen story.

The very notion of a specimen story as applied to the reading of another story is always a misreading:

This mistake exists in every form of knowledge, insofar as knowledge is nothing other than the crystallization of symbolic activity that it forgets, once constituted. In every knowledge already constituted there is thus a dimension of error, which consists in the forgetting of the creative function of truth in its nascent form. (S II.29)

Paradoxically enough, it is precisely insofar as it embodies its own forgetting that the Oedipus myth constitutes the science of psychoanalysis. And this science only takes itself complacently (non-problematically) to be a science when it in effect *forgets* the fictive, generative moment of its birth, when it forgets that it owes its creativity—the production of its knowledge—to a myth. In this respect, psychoanalysis, which treats the real by means of the symbolic, is not so different from any other science (physics, for example). There is a fictive moment at the genesis of every science, a generative fiction (a hypothesis) at the foundation of every theory.

To borrow a metaphor from physics, one could say that the fictive psychoanalytic myth is to the *science* of psychoanalysis what the Heisenberg principle is to contemporary physics: the element of mythic narrative is something like an *uncertainty principle* of psychoanalytic theory. It does not conflict with science—it generates it—so long as it is not believed to be a certainty principle. The question of science in psychoanalysis is thus, for Lacan, not a question of cognition but a question of commitment. The concomitant acknowledgment of the psychoanalytic myth is, on the other hand, not a question of complacency in myth, but a question of exigency in and beyond the myth.

Science is the drive to *go beyond*. The scientist's commitment is at once to acknowledge myth and to attempt to go beyond the myth. Only when this mythical, narrative movement of "going beyond" stops does science stop. Only when the myth is not acknowledged, and is believed to be science, does the myth prevail at the expense of science. It is precisely when we believe we are beyond the myth that we indulge in fiction. There is no *beyond* to myth—science is always, in one way or another, a new generative myth.

There is no *beyond* to the narrative movement of the myth. But the narrative movement of the myth is precisely that which always takes us—if we dare go with it—*beyond itself.*

"Many complain," writes Kafka,[13] "that the words of the wise are always merely parables and of no use in daily life, which is the only life we have":

> When the sage says, *"go beyond,"* he does not mean that we
> should cross to some actual place, which we could do anyhow
> if the labor were worth it; he means some fabulous yonder,

something unknown to us, something too that he cannot designate more precisely, and therefore cannot help us here in the very least. All these parables really set out to say merely that the incomprehensible is incomprehensible, and we know that already. But the cares we have to struggle with every day: that is a different matter.

Concerning this a man once said: Why such reluctance? If you only followed the parables you yourselves would become parables and with that be rid of all your daily cares.

Another said: I bet that is also a parable.

The first said: You have won.

The second said: But unfortunately only in parable.

The first said: No, in reality: in parable you have lost.

Note on Texts and Abbreviations

Major Published Works by Jacques Lacan

1966   *Ecrits* (Paris: Editions du Seuil).
       English edition: *Ecrits: A Selection,* translated by Alan Sheridan
       (New York: W. W. Norton & Co., 1977).

1968   "Introduction de *Scilicet*," in *Scilicet* (Lacanian periodical, official
       organ of the Ecole freudienne de Paris), no. 1 (Paris: Seuil).

1973   *Le Séminaire, livre XI: Les Quatre Concepts fondamentaux de la
       psychanalyse* (Paris: Seuil).
       English edition: *The Four Fundamental Concepts of Psychoanaly-
       sis,* edited by Jacques-Alain Miller, translated by Alan Sheridan
       (New York: Norton, 1978)

1975   *Le Séminaire, livre I: Les Ecrits techniques de Freud* (Paris:
       Seuil).

1975   *Le Séminaire, livre XX: Encore* (Paris: Seuil).

1978   *Le Séminaire, livre II: Le Moi dans la théorie de Freud et dans la
       technique psychanalytique* (Paris: Seuil).

1981   *Le Séminaire, livre III: Les Psychoses* (Paris: Seuil).

The text of Lacan's Seminars published by Editions du Seuil was established
by Jacques-Alain Miller.

Abbreviations

E	*Ecrits* (1966)
N	Norton English editions (1977, 1978) of *Ecrits* and *Séminaire XI*
Scilicet	*"Introduction de Scilicet"* (1968)
S I	*Séminaire I* (1975)
S II	*Séminaire II* (1978)
S III	*Séminaire III* (1981)
S XI	*Séminaire XI* (1973)
S XX	*Séminaire XX* (1975)
SE	*The Standard Edition of the Complete Psychological Works of Sigmund Freud,* 24 vols., edited by James Strachey (London: Hogarth Press and the Institute of Psycho-Analysis, 1953–1974).

When the reference to the original French edition of *Ecrits* (E with page number) is not followed by a reference to the Norton English edition (N with page number), the passage quoted has not been included in Norton's selection and is in my translation.

All references to the untranslated French publications of Lacan are in my translation. The abbreviation tm (translation modified) will signal my alterations of the published English translation of the work in question.

As a rule, italics in quoted passages are mine unless otherwise indicated.

Notes

Introduction

1. Jacques Lacan (1901–1981) was trained as a physician, then as a psychiatrist, and in 1932 published a dissertation on paranoia. The psychiatrist, however, was socially and intellectually much involved with the poetic and artistic circles of the surrealists, whose impact is reflected in his work. It was only later, in the course of his clinical work and of his psychiatric teaching at the Hospital Sainte-Anne (in the thirties), that Lacan was led to the writings of Freud, whose insights he later saw it as his vocation to impart to others. He wanted to restore the radicality of Freud's texts from the distortion of inaccurate translations and oversimplified dogmatizations to which they had, in his view, been subjected.

Lacan thus became both a practicing and a teaching psychoanalyst. For nearly thirty years, he gave in Paris (first at the Ecole pratique des hautes etudes, then at the Ecole normale supérieure, and finally at the Law School Auditorium) a bimonthly public Seminar. Intended for the training of analysts, the lectures made an impact far beyond the professional circles of psychoanalysis. They were enthusiastically attended not just by analysts but by writers, artists, scientists, philosophers, and intellectuals from all disciplines—and became a focus of stimulation and fascination for the whole spectrum of the French intelligentsia from the early fifties through the seventies. The publication in 1966 of Lacan's first volume of collected essays (lectures), the *Ecrits*, increased still further Lacan's prestige and audience, even though the work's poetic style was opaque and its complexity of thought demanding, not easily accessible.

Lacan is also noted, in the history of French psychoanalysis, for the political schisms he provoked. In 1964, after two successive breaks with the International Psychoanalytical Association (1953) and with the French Society of

Psychoanalysis (1963), he founded his own school—the Ecole freudienne de Paris—which kept growing and itself became an influential institution. Lacan unexpectedly chose to dissolve it in 1980, a year before his death, to prevent his own school from being consolidated, so he said, into "a new church."

Quite apart, however, from the success of scandal he enjoyed and from the fascination he exercised, Lacan has left a body of immensely rich, complex, and challenging written work, which is what this book will focus on.

2. As we know, and as we have experienced through the reading of this passage, Lacan is difficult to understand. His style, although intriguing, is disconcerting and ambiguous. But this difficulty we all share in reading Lacan should not discourage us, because it is an integral part of what he talks about: we all have difficulty with the unconscious. This is what Lacan's language makes us hear, even as we are unable to control, or grasp exactly, what the difficulty is about. Lacan speaks enigmatically. But the enigma is about us: about our own relation to the difficulty of our own unconscious; about the nontransparency between speech and the speaking subject. "Take Socrates," says Lacan: "Intervening, at every moment, there is the demonic voice. Could one maintain that the voice that guides Socrates is not Socrates himself? The relation between Socrates and his voice is no doubt an enigma" (S xi, N 258). And once again: "It is not a question of knowing whether I speak of myself in a way that conforms to what I am, but rather of knowing whether I am the same as that of which I speak" (E, N 165).

3. For an analysis of the significance of the stylistic affinity between Lacan and Mallarmé, see my *Writing and Madness: Literature/Philosophy/Psychoanalysis* (Ithaca: Cornell University Press, 1985), esp. pp. 131–134.

4. *La "Folie" dans l'oeuvre romanesque de Stendhal* (Paris: José Corti, 1971), esp. chap. 8, "*Armance* ou la parole impossible."

5. For a specification of Lacan's crucial clinical emphases concerning the analyst's role and behavior, see in particular the section entitled "The Analyst's Responsibility, or the Function of Interpretation," in Chapter 5, and the summary of Chapter 2 later in this Introduction (in the section entitled "The Structure of the Book"), particularly the two last paragraphs of that summary.

6. Thus the heated gossip about the controversiality of Lacan's behavior and personality will, for the purposes of this book, be bracketed. No matter how legitimate these questions might be in a different context, they are irrelevant to this one: they merely stand in our way of learning from Lacan. Contrary to popular opinion, I contend that, to learn from Lacan, we do not need to think it necessary to become Lacan, or to defend Lacan the person. I wish to separate the issues of the controversy from the issues of the text: when I talk about Lacan, I am referring to his text. I am naming nothing other than the insight that his work can yield for its attentive readers.

7. For the way in which the last two questions are elaborated by Lacan, see particularly Chapter 3. The first question, in its revolutions, is at stake in Chapter 5.

8. For a further development of the impossibility of application and of the difference between application and implication of psychoanalysis, see my In-

troduction, "To Open the Question," in the volume I edited: *Literature and Psychoanalysis: The Question of Reading—Otherwise* (Baltimore: Johns Hopkins Univesity Press, 1982), pp. 5–10.

1. Renewing the Practice of Reading

1. Louis Althusser and Etienne Balibar, *Lire le capital* (Paris: Petite Collection Maspéro, 1971), p. 13; my translation.

2. Richard Rorty, "Freud, Morality, and Hermeneutics," in *New Literary History*, 12 (Autumn 1980), 177.

3. Transcribed from a recording of Lacan's talk at the Kanzer Seminar, Yale University, 24 November 1975, translated by Barbara Johnson; my italics. As a rule, italics in quoted passages are mine unless otherwise indicated.

2. The Case of Poe

1. "Although Poe was not the social outcast Baudelaire conceived him to be, he was, and still is, perhaps the most thoroughly misunderstood of all American writers." Floyd Stovall, *Edgar Poe the Poet: Essays New and Old on the Man and His Work* (Charlottesville: University of Virginia Press, 1969).

2. T. S. Eliot's famous statement on Poe in his study, "From Poe to Valéry," *Hudson Review*, Autumn 1949; reprinted in *The Recognition of Edgar Allan Poe: Selected Criticism since 1829*, ed. Eric W. Carlson (Ann Arbor: University of Michigan Press, 1966), p. 205. This collection of critical essays will hereafter be cited as *Recognition*, with individual essays abbreviated as follows: P. P. Cooke, "Edgar A. Poe" (1848); T. S. Eliot, "From Poe to Valéry" (1949); T. W. Higginson, "Poe" (1879); Aldous Huxley, "Vulgarity in Literature" (1931); J. R. Lowell, "Edgar Allan Poe" (1845); C. M. Rourke, "Edgar Allan Poe" (1931); G. B. Shaw, "Edgar Allan Poe" (1909); Edmund Wilson, "Poe at Home and Abroad" (1926); Ivor Winters, "Edgar Allan Poe: A Crisis in American Obscurantism" (1937).

3. J. W. Krutch, *Edgar Allan Poe: A Study in Genius* (New York: Knopf, 1926)

4. J. M. S. Robertson, "The Genius of Poe," *Modern Quarterly*, 3 (1926); Camille Mauclair, *Le Génie d'Edgar Poe* (Paris, 1925); John Dillon, *Edgar Allan Poe: His Genius and His Character* (New York, 1911); John R. Thompson, *The Genius and Character of Edgar Allan Poe* (privately printed, 1929); Jeannet A. Marks, *Genius and Disaster: Studies in Drugs and Genius* (New York, 1925); Jean A. Alexander, "Affidavits of Genius: French Essays on Poe," *Dissertation Abstracts*, 22 (September 1961)

5. Higginson, "Poe," *Recognition*, p. 67.

6. Swinburne, letter to Sara Sigourney Rice, 9 November 1875, *Recognition*, p. 63. Mallarmé, "Scolies," in *Oeuvres complètes*, ed. H. Mondor and G. Jean-Aubry (Paris: Pléiade, 1945), p. 223; my translation. Lowell, "Edgar Allan Poe," *Recognition*, p. 11.

7. Cooke, quoting Elizabeth Barrett, in "Edgar A. Poe," *Recognition*, p. 23; original italics.

8. Shaw, "Edgar Allan Poe," *Recognition*, p. 98.

9. Eliot, "From Poe to Valéry," *Recognition*, p. 209.

10. "The Murders in the Rue Morgue," in *Edgar Allan Poe: Selected Writings,* ed. David Galloway (New York: Penguin, 1967), p. 189; hereafter cited as *Poe.*

11. Bonaparte, *Edgar Poe* (Paris: Denöel et Steele, 1933). English edition: *Life and Works of Edgar Allan Poe,* trans. John Rodker (London: Imago, 1949). All references to Marie Bonaparte will be to the English editions.

12. Lacan, "Le Séminaire sur *La Lettre volée*," in *Ecrits* (Paris: Seuil, 1966); first translated by Jeffrey Mehlman in "French Freud," *Yale French Studies,* 48 (1972). All references here to Lacan's Poe Seminar are to the *Yale French Studies* translation.

13. Edmund Wilson: "The recent revival of interest in Poe has brought to light a good deal of new information and supplied us for the first time with a serious interpretation of his personal career, but it has so far entirely neglected to explain why we should still want to read him" (*Recognition*, p. 142).

14. Mauclair, *Le Génie d'Edgar Poe;* quoted in *Poe,* p. 24.

15. Galloway, Introduction to *Poe,* pp. 24–25.

16. For a remarkable analysis of the way repetition is enacted in the problematics of reading set in motion by Lacan's text, see Barbara Johnson's "The Frame of Reference: Poe, Lacan, Derrida," in *The Critical Difference: Essays in the Rhetoric of Contemporary Criticism* (Baltimore: Johns Hopkins University Press, 1980).

17. "Need we emphasize the similarity of these two sequences? Yes, for the resemblance we have in mind is not a simple collection of traits chosen only in order to delete their difference. And it would not be enough to retain those common traits at the expense of the others for the slightest truth to result. It is rather the intersubjectivity in which the two actions are motivated that we wish to bring into relief, as well as the three terms through which it structures them. The special status of these terms results from their corresponding simultaneously to the three logical moments through which the decision is precipitated and to the three places it assigns to the subjects among whom it constitutes a choice . . . Thus three moments, structuring three glances, borne by three subjects, incarnated each time by different characters." "Seminar on *The Purloined Letter*," pp. 43–44.

18. "The Murders in the Rue Morgue," *Poe,* p. 204

19. I have attempted, however, an elementary exploration of such an approach with respect to Henry James in my essay, "Turning the Screw of Interpretation," in *Writing and Madness: Literature/Philosophy/Psychoanalysis* (Ithaca: Cornell University Press, 1985).

20. The formula is David Galloway's (*Poe,* p. 24).

3. What Difference Does Psychoanalysis Make?

1. Charles Sanders Peirce, "The Scientific Attitude and Fallibilism," in *Philosophical Writings*, ed. Justus Buchler (New York: Dover 1955), p. 58.

2. What is called for is, in Lacan's own terms, "a return to the shades" (E 411, N 123).

3. Chapter 1, p. 23.

4. It should be remembered that Copernicus' book, which reports his discovery, was entitled *On the Celestial Revolutions*.

4. Psychoanalysis and Education

1. Plato, *Meno* 70a, 71a, 82a, trans. G. M. A. Grube (Indianapolis: Hackett Publishing Company, 1980), pp. 3, 14.

2. For Lacan "teaching" involves "the relationship of the individual to language" (E 445).

3. Anna Freud, *Psychoanalysis for Teachers and Parents*, trans. Barbara Low (Boston: Beacon Press, 1960), pp. 95–96.

4. Ibid., p. 105.

5. Catherine Millot, interview in *L'Ane, le magasine freudien*, 1 (April–May 1981), 19.

6. Catherine Millot, *Freud anti-pedagogue* (Paris: Bibliotheque d'Ornicar, 1979).

7. As soon as analytic knowledge *is* exchanged, it ceases to be knowledge and becomes opinion: "the sum of prejudices that every knowledge contains, and that each of us transports . . . Knowledge is always, somewhere, only one's belief that one knows" (S II.56).

8. Sophocles, *Oedipus the King*, trans. David Grene, in *Complete Greek Tragedies*, vol. 1, ed. David Grene and Richmond Lattimore (Chicago: University of Chicago Press, 1954), pp. 25–26.

9. The therapeutic analysis of patients is "interminable" to the extent that repression can never be totally lifted, only displaced. See Freud's letter to Fliess, dated 16 April 1900: " 'E's career as a patient has at last come to an end . . . His riddle is *almost* completely solved, his condition is excellent . . . At the moment a residue of this symptoms remains. I am beginning to understand that the apparently interminable nature of the treatment is something determined by law and is dependent on the transference." Hence Freud speaks of "the asymptotic terminaton of treatment" (SE 23.215; original italics).

10. Lacan's occasional master's pose in his seminars—however mystifying to the audience—invariably exhibits itself as a parodic symptom of the analysand.

11. Plato, *Apology*, 22a-c, in *Dialogues of Plato*, trans. Benjamin Jowett (New York: Washington Square Press, 1973), p. 12.

12. "There is," writes Freud, "at least one spot in every dream at which it is unplumbable—a navel, as it were, that is the point of contact with the unknown" (SE 4.111).

13. Nietzsche, *Thus Spoke Zarathustra*, trans. Walter Kaufmann, in *The Portable Nietzsche* (New York: Viking, 1971), p. 239.

5. Beyond Oedipus

1. Roy Schafer, "Narration in the Psychoanalytic Dialogue," in *The Analytic Attitude* (New York: Basic Books, 1983), pp. 218–219.

2. Freud, letter to Wilhelm Fliess, 15 October 1897, in *The Origins of Psychoanalysis,* trans. Eric Mosbacher and James Strachey (New York: Basic Books, 1954), pp. 221–224.

3. Melanie Klein, "The Importance of Symbol-Formation in the Development of the Ego" (1930), in her *Contributions to Psycho-Analysis, 1921–1945* (New York: Hillary House, 1948), pp. 236–250.

4. See "The Mirror-Stage as Formative of the Function of the I as Revealed in Psychoanalytic Experience" (E 93–100, N 1–7).

5. See E 277–278, N 66–67: "Even when in fact it is represented by a single person, the paternal function concentrates in itself both imaginary and real relations, always more or less inadequate to the symbolic relation which constitutes it. It is in the name of the father that we must recognize the support of the symbolic function which, from the dawn of history, has identified his person with the figure of the law."

6. I am using the term "performative" as established by J. L. Austin in *Philosophical Papers* (New York: Oxford University Press, 1970) and *How To Do Things with Words* (Cambridge: Harvard University Press, 1975). For a different, complementary perspective on the relation between speech acts and psychoanalysis (as well as on the theoretical relation between Austin and Lacan), see my *The Literary Speech-Act: Don Juan with J. L. Austin, or Seduction in Two Languages,* trans. Catherine Porter (Ithaca: Cornell University Press, 1983); original edition in French, *Le Scandale du corps parlant: Don Juan avec Austin, ou La Séduction en deux langues* (Paris: Seuil, 1980).

7. Shafer, p. 218. Even though Schafer's account of "Narration in the Psychoanalytic Dialogue" is very different from Lacan's, it is remarkable in its own right, reaching the complexity and subtlety of psychoanalytic insight by a different pathway. It is only at the opening of his inquiry that Schafer seems to hold the commonsensical view of psychoanalytic dialogue, of which Lacan's more paradoxical, radical approach challenges precisely the common sense. But Schafer's own study in effect unsettles, through infinite refinement and subtle complications, the commonsensical description that is its starting point. As Schafer himself puts it, "psychoanalysis does not take common sense plain but rather transforms it into a comprehensive distillate"; and "more than one such distillation of common sense has been offered in the name of psychoanalysis" (p. 214). No more than Lacan's, Schafer's own creative psychoanalytic thinking does not take common sense plain.

8. Sophocles, *Oedipus at Colonus,* trans. E. F. Walting, in *The Theban Plays* (Baltimore: Penguin Classics, 1947; reprinted 1965), scene 2, p. 83.

9. Sophocles, *Oedipus at Colonus,* trans. David Grene, in *Complete Greek Tragedies,* vol. 1, ed. David Grene and Richmond Lattimore (Chicago: University

of Chicago Press, 1954), scene 2, p. 96. Subsequent quotations from *Oedipus at Colonus* will refer to this edition, by scene and page number.

10. This insight was first suggested to me (in a course on the Oedipus myth) by a student, Teddy Cohn, to whom I here address this purloined letter of thanks.

11. E 415. See also above, Chapter 3, pp. 61–66.

12. Aboard the ship that transported him to the United States to give the Clark lectures, Freud apparently said to Jung (who reported it to Lacan): "They don't know that we bring with us the Plague."

13. Franz Kafka, "On Parables," in *Parables and Paradoxes* (New York: Schocken Books, 1970), p. 11.

Printed in the United States
203479BV00004B/55-66/A